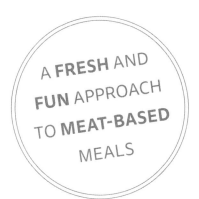

A **FRESH** AND **FUN** APPROACH TO **MEAT-BASED** MEALS

MW01070985

carnivore *in the* kitchen

COURTNEY LUNA

VICTORY BELT PUBLISHING INC.

LAS VEGAS

Cover design, interior design, and illustrations by Yordan Terziev and Boryana Yordanova

Cover and lifestyle photography by Camryn Clair

Printed in Canada

TC 0124

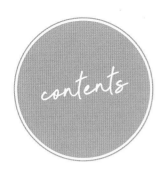

contents

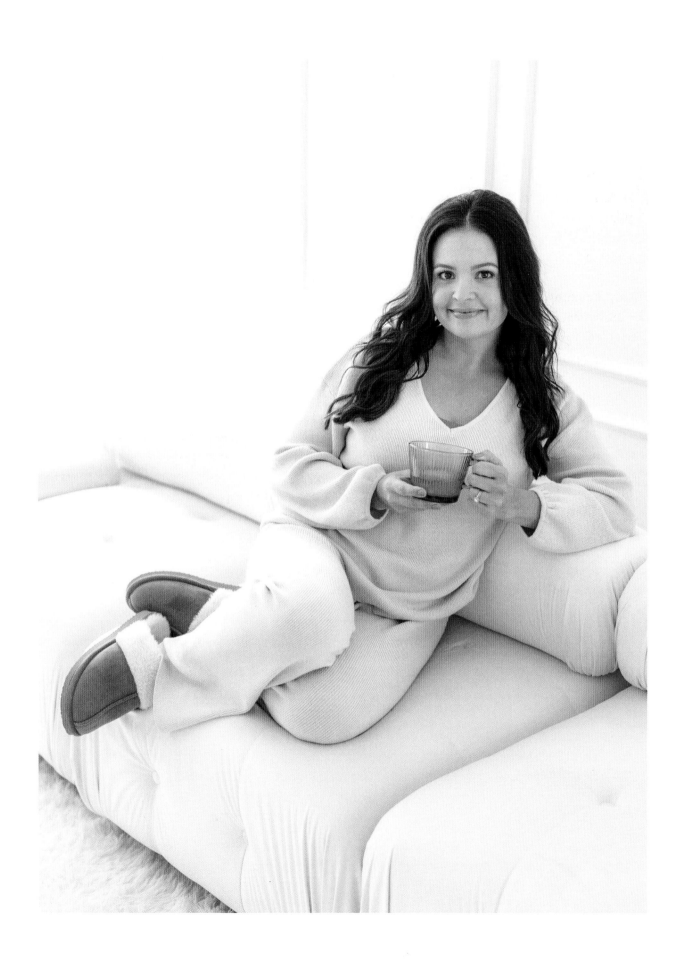

acknowledgments

A huge thank you to my meaty community who "Eat Meat + Question Everything." I appreciate all the love, support, and sticking up for me in the comments. This book was able to come to fruition because of you!

To my amazing recipe testers. Thank you for the honest feedback to get these recipes perfected. Taking the time to make these and give me your honest opinion means the world!

To the best book crew ever. Emmie, thank you for discovering me, and thanks to Lance for taking a chance on me. Pam and Holly, thank you for being kind and patient with me while I figured out how to get what I do in the kitchen down on paper. Yordan, Boryana, Justin, and Kat, thank you for making this book look so beautiful! Susan, I just love your energy, and I appreciate all your ideas and help to get this book out there!

To my friends and extended family. Thank you for checking in with me and for all your encouragement during this project.

And finally, to my family. Thank you to my beautiful kiddos, Archer and Hazel, for being the best little recipe testers. Even though it was stressful at times, I'm so happy we have the memories of all of us together while I was testing and photographing the recipes. To all four of my parents and my in-laws for supporting the recipe testing, entertaining the kids, and cheering me on. To my mom, Gma, for being an extension of me and for helping me take care of the kids so I could get this dream project done. And to my favorite person, my husband, Jeff. Thank you for being my therapist, my right-hand man, and my rock. For brainstorming ideas, taste testing, and washing dishes. You deserve a medal for putting up with me the last seven months. Well, the last eleven years, really. I love you.

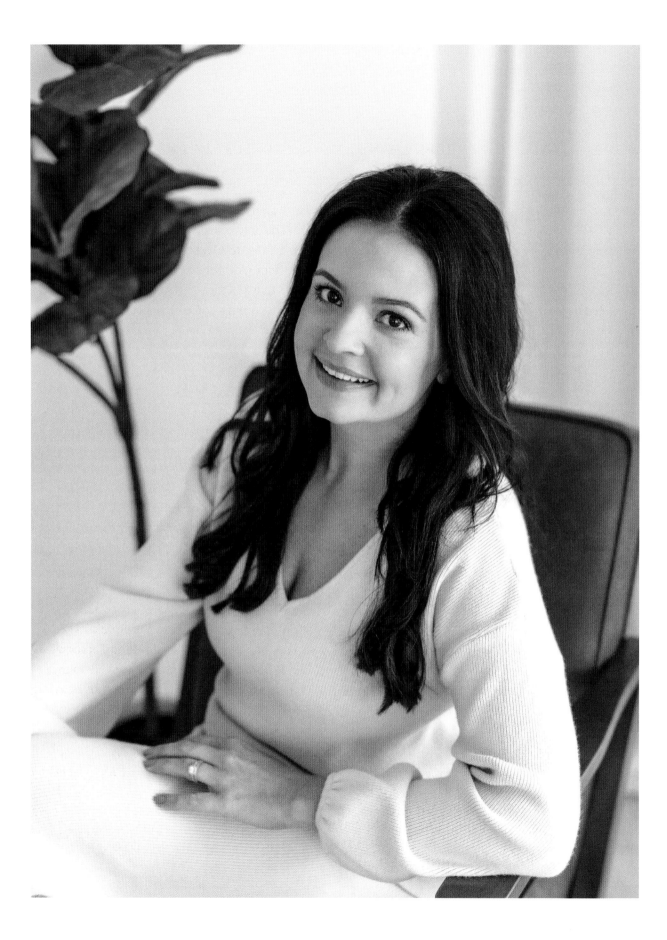

my story

I've always had a love for food and cooking. Watching the Food Network with a glass (or bottle) of wine on a Friday night was my idea of a good time. If you had told me years ago that today I would be cooking with only meat and animal products—and be sober—I would not have believed it.

It's weird to me that this is how I eat now because I spent years cooking both as a hobby and for work, and everything I made had a ton of ingredients. My passion for cooking really grew when I became a yacht stewardess in 2010 and began working closely with the chefs on board. That's where it all began! I learned so much, not only about food preparation and recipe development but also that being a chef is way more fun than scrubbing toilets and serving cocktails on the aft deck. Joke's on me, because my first cooking gig was as a chef/stewardess, so I still had to scrub toilets and serve the guests in addition to cooking all the meals.

I owe a lot to my time spent working on yachts, and the people I worked with. In late 2013, my chef at the time, Kelley, hooked me up with a boat back home in Newport Beach, California. Not only was I eager to be closer to Jeff (my now-husband whom I met early 2013) and be done with long-distance dating, but I was ready to cook for a living. Leaving that boat was difficult because both the owners and the crew were amazing (hi, Indiscretion fam!), but I knew it was time to move on.

My first official cooking gig was on this new boat. I was crew chef/stewardess, and it was a dream job. Even though I still had stewardess duties, it was wonderful to cook for everyone too. The only reason I left is because the boat was headed to Alaska, and I wasn't ready to be away from Jeff for six months. (Do I sound like a stage-five clinger yet?) Anyhoo, I decided then that I was going to dive into the chef side of the yachting world full-time.

I became a freelance yacht chef, and thanks to referrals, word of mouth, and crew agents, I was able to have a very successful career for four years. Being flown out to a Caribbean island, cooking for the owners and crew on the charter trip, and then flying back home was a wonderful experience. The meals I prepared were typical Standard American Diet, lots of meat, potatoes, and veggies, but in a fancy way. Desserts were served after every dinner, pastries for breakfast, and cookies at tea time. I really enjoyed cooking that way. Sugar really makes people happy and that was how I showed my love . . . with a killer Snickers pie, a decadent sweet corn casserole, and epic twice-baked potatoes. When guests arrived on my charter, they probably left five pounds heavier. While those foods were delicious, I'm horrified by how I used to eat, knowing what I know now. Over all those years, I never had a good relationship with food. I thought I did because I loved food and was obsessed with it, but I didn't realize how much it controlled me.

The yacht chef chapter ended in 2017 when I left the industry to become a mom, and soon after I decided to start sharing my cooking adventures and recipes online. At the time I was following a low-carb diet and dabbling in keto. All my low-carb recipes were well received, never a bad comment. Imagine my surprise when my focus shifted to carnivore... that's when my social media platforms took off and people began to express opinions about what I was posting.

The shift in the content I posted online was born out of necessity. I'd discovered that going low carb and even keto was helpful but not the solution for me. I'd been a yo-yo dieter for twenty-five years, and it wasn't until I adopted the carnivore lifestyle that I understood why. Just like an alcoholic can't moderate their drinking, I can't moderate my carb and sugar intake. I need to abstain completely. One donut would lead to the whole dozen. Or, if I was able to eat just one, I would think about donuts for the rest of the day. The mental hold that food had over me was exhausting—I faced either a vicious cycle of binging and restricting or I was trying to fit foods that didn't serve me well, like donuts and ice cream, into my macros. Then I heard my friend Serena talk about abstainers versus moderators. Figuring out that I am an abstainer, not a moderator, was life-changing for me. Knowing this keeps me on track because I understand I am one bite away from slipping back to my old ways. Now it makes sense why all the diets I tried (Weight Watchers, SlimFast, Paleo, and keto) didn't work: because they allowed me to have sugar. Even artificial sweeteners continued the sugar cravings for me. (To read more about food freedom and about abstainers versus moderators, see the discussion on page 16.)

Now, you might be wondering why I don't at least eat non-sweet-tasting vegetables, then? I will dive into that subject later, in chapter 1, but for now I will just say that they cause gas and irritate my gut, and besides, rib eyes are so much tastier than broccoli.

It was my husband who discovered animal-based nutrition and spent a month sending me Dr. Paul Saladino's videos, without comment. Dr. Saladino promotes an animal-based diet, which includes meat, organs, fruit, honey and raw dairy—no veggies. One day I asked my husband why he was sending me those clips. Did he really think we shouldn't be eating vegetables? I thought the idea was crazy! Jeff said he was going to investigate it. He took a deep dive into the content Dr. Ken Berry, Dr. Anthony Chaffee, and Dr. Shawn Baker were sharing online, along with the work of other influencers in the carnivore space—Kelly Hogan, Lillie Kane, and Bella Ma (aka Steak and Butter Gal), to name a few. I was coming off of what essentially was a four-month eating binge and was willing to try anything that might give me my life back. On May 10, 2022, we decided to dive in, and the rest is history!

Jeff started out strict carnivore, while I opted for animal based, which allows some fruit in addition to animal products. (You can find more information about the various carnivore eating styles on page 14.) My carb-addicted self was not ready to give up sweets, even if it was just in fruit form. After five weeks, I did feel better overall, but I noticed that even after eating a huge meal, my mouth still wanted blueberries. Although I was full and didn't need any more food, sweet flavors still lured me in. That's when I realized I had to ditch fruit entirely and go strict carnivore.

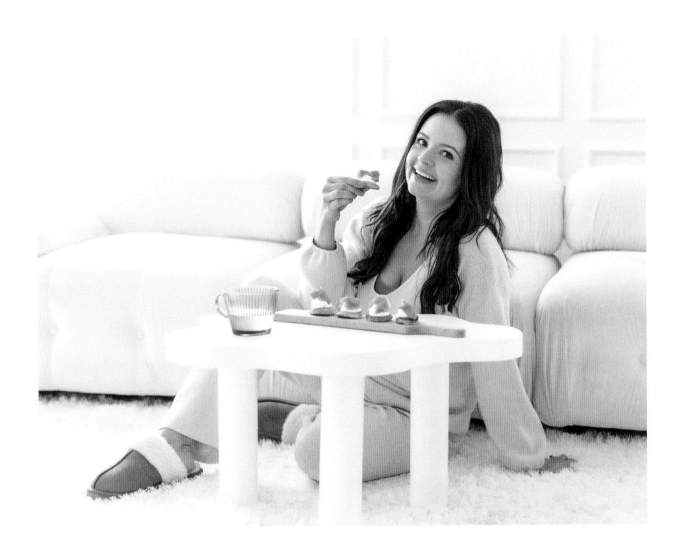

In less than a year of eating only meat, seafood, eggs, and dairy, I lost 45 pounds. My acne cleared up, I went off my medication for anxiety and depression, I had mental freedom around food, I had tons of energy, my lab work had improved, and I had zero gas or bloating. I just felt amazing.

For all these reasons and more, I am passionate about this way of eating, and no matter the amount of hate I receive on social media (and if you follow me on TikTok, you know I get a lot), I will never let it silence me. It has become my mission to help spread the word about carnivore. People are changing their lives by eating this way. I have seen so many success stories from individuals who have healed from health problems such as autoimmune issues, type 2 diabetes, high blood pressure, skin conditions, infertility, polycystic ovary syndrome (PCOS), and many more. If you have any sort of ache, pain, or health issue, I recommend giving carnivore a shot.

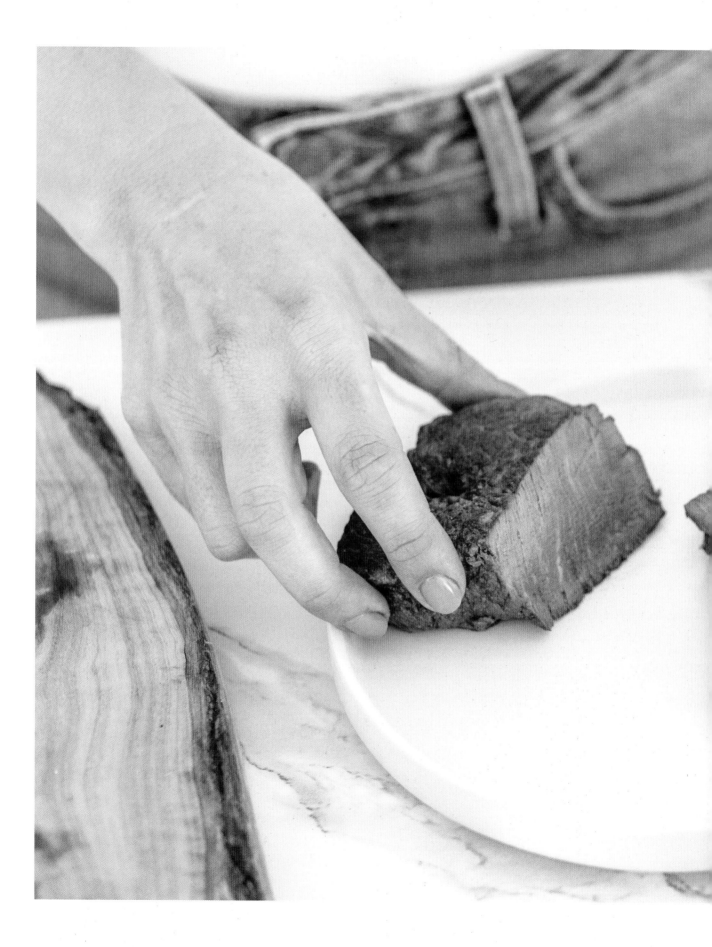

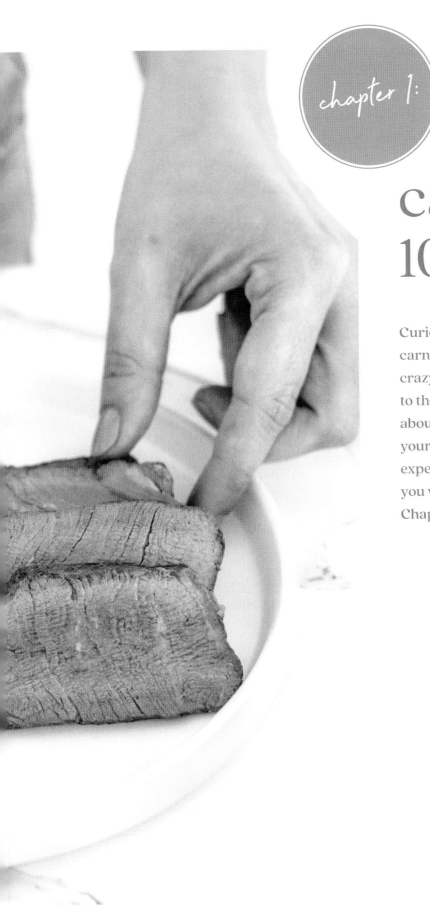

chapter 1:

carnivore 101

Curious about how to get started on the carnivore diet—or why anyone would be crazy enough to eat this way? You've come to the right place. In this chapter, I talk about making the transition and equipping your kitchen for success. If you're already experienced with meat-based eating and you want to skip straight to the recipes in Chapter 3, that's fine, too.

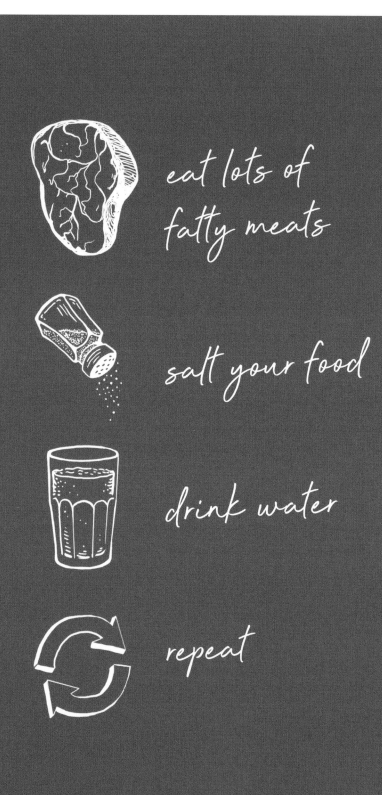

eat lots of fatty meats

salt your food

drink water

repeat

starting your carnivore journey

Most people turn to the carnivore diet either for weight loss or because they have health issues. They've typically tried everything else and finally come to this "extreme" diet because nothing else has worked. Does this sound like you? If it does, carnivore could be the right choice for you. Not only does it work wonders for weight loss, but it can also help you get your health back.

Eating this way is the ultimate elimination diet. We can't thrive on eating only carrots, but we can thrive on eating only beef. It provides all the micronutrients we need. Eating this way also brings together like-minded people because we're going against the grain. And once you realize we've been lied to about nutrition (for example, we're told that red meat causes heart disease, butter is bad, and we need vegetables to survive), you start to question everything else you've been told.

If you're looking to jump right into a meat-based way of eating, the shortest how-to I can give you is this:

Eat lots of fatty meats, salt your food, drink water, repeat.

There's a lot more that can go into it, but try not to let it overwhelm you. There's also nothing wrong with easing into a carnivore diet; while I (and many others) started cold turkey, you can go slowly, gradually lowering your carbs, increasing your protein intake, ditching the sugar and seed oils, and so on.

the types of meat-based diets

Let's begin by breaking down the most common variations of a meat-based diet:

Red meat (beef, pork, lamb), organ meats, poultry, seafood, eggs, dairy, and salt.
You can drink coffee or tea and/or use seasonings other than salt if you tolerate them. This is the most common, or standard, version of the carnivore diet.

Only meats and fats from ruminant animals, plus salt.
Examples of ruminant meats are beef, bison, lamb, goat, and venison. This stricter version of carnivore is a great place to start if you are looking to use it as an elimination diet. After a period of eating a lion diet, you can try slowly adding other foods back in if you wish.

All animals, organs, animal products (such as dairy and eggs), fruit, maple syrup, honey, and salt.
Coffee, tea, and seasonings other than salt can be included if you tolerate them. Note that the fruit category here includes avocados, coconut, olives, cucumbers, and squashes; these foods, though commonly thought of as vegetables, are in fact botanically classified as fruits and are permitted on an animal-based diet. If you go animal based, I suggest keeping carbs low for best results.

Beef, bacon, butter, and eggs. Salt is allowed, along with spices at your discretion. And of course, coffee and tea get a free pass. This acronym was coined by Dr. Ken Berry, a prominent advocate for meat-based diets, and a lot of people use it as a reset or a monthly challenge. It's a simple way to quickly get some weight off and improve your insulin sensitivity without having to worry about tracking macros (protein, carbs, and fat). Some people feel their best eating this way, but I find that after a few weeks, my body begins to crave other animal foods, particularly chicken wings and salmon.

Meat-heavy like the previous examples, but allows some low-carb fruits and vegetables while keeping carbohydrates low to maintain a ketogenic ("keto") diet. Keto involves maintaining a state of ketosis, where your body burns fat instead of glucose for energy. To do so, you typically need to eat less than 30 grams of total (not net) carbs per day. You can consume coffee, tea, and seasonings other than salt at your discretion if you tolerate them. Some keto sweeteners, such as stevia and monkfruit, along with low-carb flours like almond and coconut, are also allowed if well tolerated, but I suggest you stay focused on meats, fats, and some low-carb fruit or vegetables. (To read more about managing macros, see pages 20 to 21.)

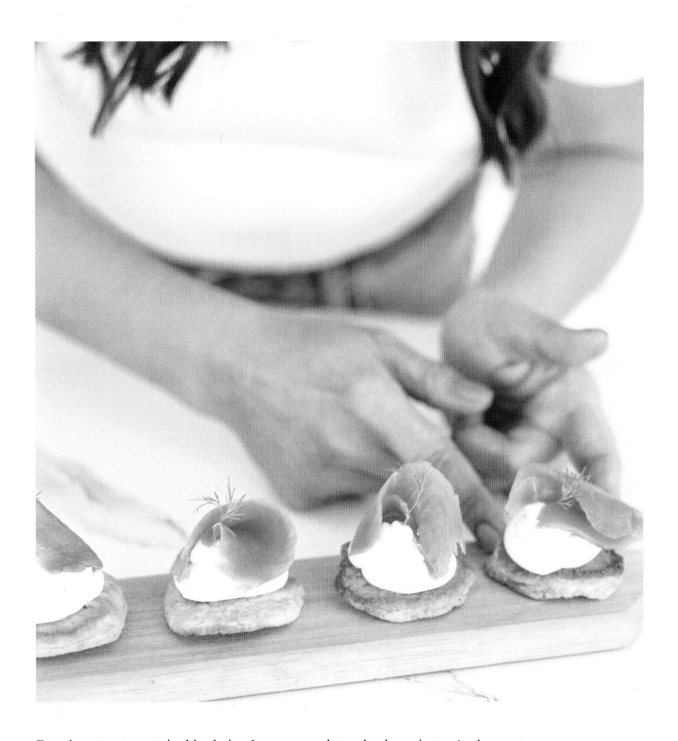

For a long-term, sustainable choice, I recommend standard carnivore. As the most nutrient-dense and nutritionally complete meat, beef is what we should prioritize, but "eating the rainbow" of animal foods is a smart idea because pork, poultry, seafood, and other meats provide nutrients that beef doesn't, such as the omega-3s in fish. Try playing around with the different variations of carnivore to see how each one makes you feel. I normally eat standard carnivore but also like to play around with monthly BBBE challenges when my dairy consumption starts to get out of hand.

the benefits of eating this way

For anyone who is interested, I recommend giving the carnivore diet a shot for thirty days—ninety days would be even better. Something magical happens at that three-month mark. Things you didn't even realize were an issue—that you tolerated as being "normal"—are likely to go away, and you'll be surprised by how great you feel. (Note that any of the first four versions of carnivore listed in the previous section will work for a thirty-day or three-month reset. Since ketovore includes plant foods, it's not ideal as a reset diet.)

Benefits you may see include increased energy, improved mental health, weight loss, clearer skin, improved digestion, elimination of gas or bloating, and stronger hair and nails. A meat-based diet can also help with autoimmune issues, irritable bowel syndrome (IBS), ulcerative colitis, Hashimoto's, polycystic ovarian syndrome (PCOS), and so much more. People have drastically changed their lives for the better by eating this way. In Dr. Berry's words, this is the "Proper Human Diet."

Another key benefit of the carnivore diet is that it can help you heal your relationship with food. The mental freedom that this streamlined way of eating brings is life-changing. Knowing whether you are an abstainer or moderator when it comes to food can also really help you stay on track and remember your "why" for eating this way. To figure out which one you are, think back to past habits. Can you occasionally have a treat or a cheat meal and then get back on track without giving it another thought? Then you are a moderator. But if eating that treat or cheat meal causes you to obsess about having another treat or cheat meal or leads to a binge, then you are an abstainer, and you need to abstain from foods that make you feel that way and have a hold over you.

I know it doesn't entirely make sense because carnivore is the ultimate elimination diet, but removing foods that don't make you feel good mentally or physically will change your perspective on eating. Since I started following the standard carnivore diet, I no longer have cravings or desires for other foods. I don't think about how I can fit that slice of cake into my macros or how I can have just a little dessert and not binge on the whole thing, and I don't binge on the dessert anyway and then restrict the next day—a vicious cycle. No dessert tastes as good as finally being free from that mentality. Food no longer has a hold on me. This is why I choose to omit something as innocent-sounding as fruit from my diet—because the sugar in the fruit would have power over me, and I would eat more fruit because it's sweet and not because I was hungry.

why meat is good for you

The consumption of meat, especially within the frameworks of the carnivore and ketogenic diets, has many health benefits, primarily due to the nutrient density and quality of animal foods. Meat is a powerhouse of essential nutrients, providing high-quality protein, amino acids, essential fatty acids, and vitamins and minerals. All are crucial for muscle maintenance, immune function, and overall health.

• **AMINO ACIDS:** Amino acids are the building blocks of protein. Meat contains all nine essential amino acids necessary for the human body's growth and repair. These amino acids are termed "essential" because our bodies cannot synthesize them; they must be obtained from our diet. High-quality protein supports muscle growth, repair, and maintenance, which is particularly important for physical health and recovery.

• **ESSENTIAL FATTY ACIDS:** Meats, especially from fish and grass-fed animals, are abundant sources of omega-3 fatty acids. These fats are crucial for brain health and reducing inflammation, and they have been linked to a lower risk of heart disease.

• **VITAMINS AND MINERALS:** Meat is rich in B vitamins (particularly B12), zinc, selenium, iron, and phosphorus. Vitamin B12, found naturally only in animal products, is vital for nerve function and the production of DNA and red blood cells. Iron from meat (heme iron) is more easily absorbed by the body than iron from plant sources, making it crucial for preventing anemia.

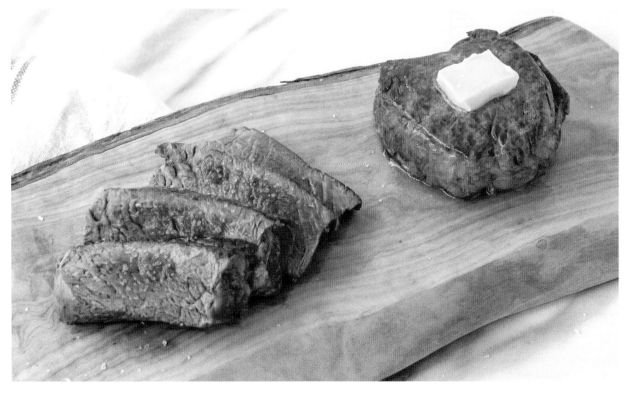

why plant foods can be harmful

The idea that vegetables can be harmful may seem baffling given that we're told vegetables are a fundamental part of a healthy diet. But eating plant foods isn't all it's cracked up to be.

Plants can't run away from the creatures who wish to eat them, so they produce defense chemicals to protect themselves, notably lectins, oxalates, and phytates. These substances are meant to prevent animals from eating the plants, and some experts say that they are not good for us humans to ingest, either.

• **LECTINS** are a type of protein found in many plant foods, mainly grains and legumes. They can bind to the digestive tract lining and disrupt the absorption of nutrients. Some lectins may also stimulate an immune response, leading to inflammatory reactions and gastrointestinal discomfort in sensitive individuals.

• **OXALATES** are found in many plant foods, including leafy greens, vegetables, fruits, nuts, and seeds. While a moderate intake of oxalate-containing foods is safe for most people, excessive consumption can lead to health issues. High levels of oxalates can contribute to the formation of kidney stones, particularly in individuals who are prone to them. Oxalates can also bind to important minerals such as calcium, reducing their bioavailability and potentially leading to nutrient deficiencies.

• **PHYTATES** are found in whole grains, legumes, seeds, and some nuts. They can bind to minerals such as iron, zinc, magnesium, and calcium, making those nutrients less absorbable in the digestive tract. This can potentially lead to mineral deficiencies, especially in individuals whose diets are heavily plant-based and who do not get enough of these minerals from other sources.

However, fruit gets a pass for some who eat carnivore since it is the least toxic part of the plant. Fruit is actually meant to attract consumption. Typically bright, aromatic, and pretty-looking, fruit encourages birds and other critters to eat it, which safeguards the rest of the plant and helps the plant reproduce. That being said, if you are not a moderator (refer to page 16), I would keep fruit out of your diet. The fructose can cause you to crave sugar.

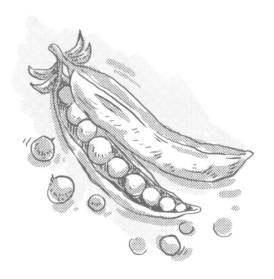

the importance of electrolytes

The maintenance of the electrolytes sodium, magnesium, and potassium is very important on a low-carb diet such as carnivore or keto, more so in the beginning when transitioning from a higher-carb way of eating. Transitioning to a low-carb diet can lead to significant shifts in fluid and electrolyte balance. When carbohydrates are restricted, the body begins to burn through glycogen stores (stored glucose) for energy, which also releases the water bound to it. This can lead to a rapid loss of water and electrolytes in the first few weeks, known as the "keto flu," with symptoms including fatigue, headache, and muscle cramps. You may wish to supplement these three key electrolytes, but many people thrive without doing so. Sodium is an easy one; simply salt your food! Magnesium and potassium are found in meats, but you could also supplement with electrolyte drinks or capsules.

• **SODIUM:** Salt your food liberally to your enjoyment. You can add a pinch of salt to a glass of water, too—just not too much or you will find yourself running to the bathroom. A bit of salt on your tongue can also help with any sugar cravings you may be having.

• **MAGNESIUM:** Many people are deficient in magnesium no matter what type of diet they eat. This electrolyte has wonderful health benefits, from alleviating anxiety to reducing leg cramps. It is available as a supplement in multiple forms: magnesium glycinate helps ease anxiety and pain and supports sleep, while magnesium citrate is great for those having constipation issues. Beef, pork, chicken, turkey, anchovies, and salmon are good food sources of magnesium.

• **POTASSIUM:** This electrolyte gets less attention than magnesium and sodium, but it's still something to pay attention to. It is included in electrolyte drinks and supplements, but you can also get it from bacon. Best news ever! Other meats that provide substantial amounts of potassium are chicken, beef, and pork.

putting fears about vitamin C to rest

Based on what we are taught about food, it's logical to assume that people who follow a carnivore diet—devoid of plants and fruit—are not getting enough vitamin C. But there is more to it than that. When you are on a low-carb diet, you may require less vitamin C because it is not competing with glucose for absorption in your body.

The relationship between vitamin C and glucose is a fascinating example of how dietary composition can influence nutrient requirements. Vitamin C and glucose share a similar chemical structure and compete for uptake by cells through the same transport mechanisms. In a diet that's high in carbohydrates, glucose can inhibit the absorption of vitamin C, potentially increasing the body's requirement for this essential nutrient. Conversely, in a low-carb diet where glucose intake is minimal, such as carnivore or

keto, this competitive inhibition is significantly reduced. Because the body can absorb and utilize vitamin C more efficiently, it may require less of this vitamin.

In addition, without the oxidative stress brought on by metabolizing large amounts of carbohydrates, the body may require less vitamin C for antioxidant protection. Furthermore, some experts argue that a diet rich in animal products provides sufficient vitamin C for the body's needs in the absence of carbohydrates, as historical evidence suggests that populations thriving on meat-heavy diets did not suffer from vitamin C deficiency. To sum up, the trace amounts of vitamin C found in muscle meats are enough to ward off scurvy. Organ meats, though not required as part of a carnivore diet, are a particularly good source of vitamin C and are very nutritious in general.

tracking your macros

Many people can eat when they're hungry and stop when they're full, while others have a hard time listening to their hunger cues. Tracking macros is a handy tool and can be especially helpful when you begin eating a carnivore diet. If you're coming from a place of undereating, having a visual of an ideal amount of food may help you feel permitted to eat what your body needs without fear. If you're coming from a place of overeating, it's equally helpful to have a visual of the amount you should be eating while your hunger cues sort themselves out.

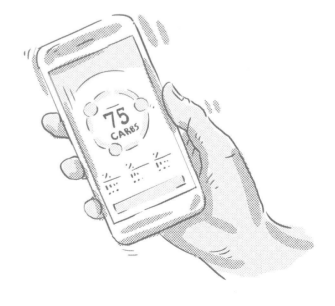

Essentially, tracking macros involves counting the number of grams of protein and fat you consume each day. (Because a meat-based diet is naturally low in carbohydrates, carbs are less of a concern here.) For standard carnivore, a good place to start is to take your goal weight and eat that number of grams of fat and protein each day. If your goal weight is 130 pounds, for example, you would aim for 130 grams of protein and 130 grams of fat. This is just a guideline, and you may want to adjust these numbers to your individual needs. Some people feel better when they increase their protein intake and lower their fat intake a bit, while others may feel better lowering the protein a bit and upping the fat. The basic ratio of equal parts fat and protein helped me lose 45 pounds, but to get through my weight loss stall and lose an additional 10 pounds, I ended up upping my protein intake a bit and lowering the fat. Hormones can come into play and affect your macro needs, too. Everyone is different, and your macros may vary from day to day.

If you follow a ketovore diet, your macros typically would be the same as for standard carnivore but would allow for up to 20 to 30 grams of total—not net—carbs per day. But everyone reacts differently, and you can play around with your carb intake and test your ketone levels using a ketone meter or test strips to see what your maximum amount of carbs is to stay in ketosis.

For animal based, you would keep your protein intake similar to standard carnivore but lower your fat intake to allow for more carbs. I suggest not going over 75 to 100 grams of total carbs per day, staying in a range that is still considered low carb.

adjusting to a meat-based diet

The first week of your carnivore diet, you may not be as hungry as you were before. Eating mostly meat is very satiating. Don't force yourself to eat if you're not hungry, but be aware of this possibility if you find that you tend to undereat consistently.

You might experience low-carb flu symptoms such as nausea, headaches, and fatigue, which can also affect your appetite. Just eat what you can, get your electrolytes, and stay hydrated.

As your body adjusts, you will find that your hunger levels even out and that any keto flu symptoms will resolve themselves. For me, this took a few days; typically, this adjustment period ranges from a few days to a couple weeks.

sorting out poop issues

Poop is one of the topics that I get asked about most frequently, and, gross as it is, it's one of my favorite topics to talk about. I apologize for including poop talk in a cookbook, but since it's directly related to how and what you're eating, I feel it's necessary.

Many people have loose stools or constipation in the beginning stages of eating a carnivore diet. If you have loose stools, the cause is the increased fat that you're consuming. In this case, I would stay away from liquid rendered fat. If you're browning ground beef, for example, avoid the fatty liquid it releases until your body has adapted to your new diet. Drain the meat well. Stick to hard, solid fats—solid butter, tallow, and cheese—or sour cream. Give your digestive system all the help you can.

While you're adapting is not the best time to do intermittent fasting. That would require you to eat too much fat at once and contribute to the loose stools problem. Instead, spread out your eating over three meals. Chew your food as thoroughly as you can, letting your saliva break it down, which will make less work for your stomach. Try not to drink much during your meals, as the liquid can dilute your stomach acid. Just know that it will get better, and in the meantime, always know where the nearest bathroom is.

If you are experiencing constipation, on the other hand, do the opposite: Eat lots of fat, incorporating the liquid fat. Make sure you stay hydrated, and try taking magnesium citrate, which can act as a natural laxative.

using meal plans

Weekly meal plans can be a practical tool, no matter your style of eating. But when first acquainting yourself with a new diet, they can be indispensable. To ease you into this way of eating, I've included three week-long plans in this book: Standard Carnivore, Dairy-Free Carnivore, and Lion Diet (see pages 46 to 53). Shopping lists are provided as well to make everything as easy as possible.

I recommend trying all three plans to see how you feel and determine which version suits your body best. It may be easier to slowly work your way into the most restrictive version so you're not going cold turkey—pun intended. To do that, start with Standard Carnivore, which includes dairy; then go dairy-free; and finally try the Lion Diet meal plan.

key ingredients

Now that you have an idea of what carnivore is and how to get started, let's talk about ingredients. A lot of people think this way of eating is expensive, but please don't let cost scare you away from trying it; if you're on a budget, it can be done very cheaply. (See the "Shopping Tips" sidebar on the next page for suggestions.) A lot of people say that eliminating all of the non-carnivore foods they used to buy, such as packaged snacks and bags of spring mix that inevitably end up rotting in the fridge, has cut their grocery budget in half.

While any animal or animal product qualifies as carnivore, the lists that follow will give you some parameters for when you are shopping. Note that not all of these foods are used in the recipes in this book; some are included to give you ideas for what else you can eat in this diet.

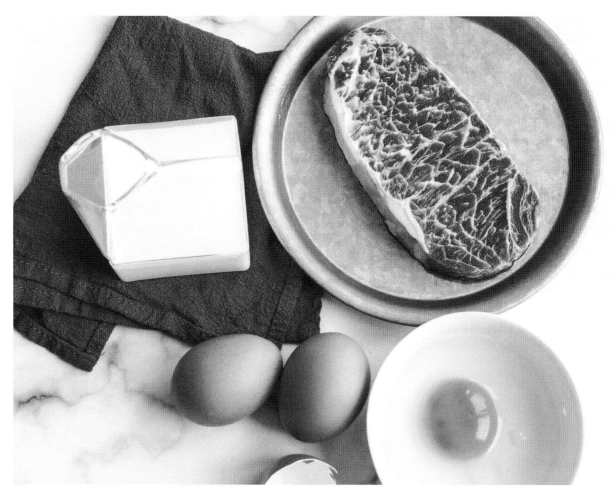

To save money and ensure quality, consider buying directly from a local farm. This way, you know where your meat is coming from. If you have the freezer space, look into purchasing a portion of a cow. Buying in bulk is almost always less expensive than buying individual cuts. While some people argue that grass-fed/-finished beef is the only way to go, grain-finished beef is just as nutritious and, in my opinion, more delicious. Though grass-finished beef does contain more omega-3s than grain-finished, I find that those extra omega-3s can give it a fishy taste. I get my beef from a small family farm that allows the cattle they raise to live their best lives, roaming around eating grass, but finishes them on grain, resulting in the most delicious beef.

Grocery store meat is very nutritious as well. Walmart has huge tubes of ground beef that can sometimes be purchased for just $2.99 a pound, which means you can eat for just $3 to $6 a day. While pasture-raised chickens fed a corn- and soy-free diet are great, the meat and eggs that they produce are expensive. Eating cheap chicken and eggs from the grocery store is still super nutritious and way better than eating a Standard American Diet.

Another way to cut costs is to shop the sales. Your local grocery likely discounts certain meats every week, and you can plan your weekly menu around those, or buy in bulk, portion, and freeze for later use.

Prioritizing beef is ideal, but all meats are nutritious, and pork and chicken are generally less expensive than beef. Most people are not eating pricey rib eyes every day, myself included!

If you're looking for a small farm to order from, here are some of my favorite farms that ship their meat to individual customers. They also share about their animals on their social media, which is cool to see.

- **BEEF:** D&D Beef (Nebraska) and Beutler Beef (Nebraska)
- **PORK:** Ancestral Farms (Iowa)
- **SUSTAINABLY FARMED SALMON (which is often more budget-friendly than wild-caught salmon):** Kvarøy Arctic (Norway). Their salmon can be purchased online from Thrive Market and is typically available at the counter at Whole Foods Market. You can find other markets that sell Kvarøy Arctic salmon near you on their website.

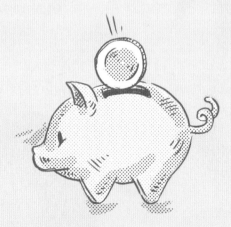

meats

- Bacon
- Beef marrow bones
- Beef roasts (brisket, chuck)
- Beef steaks (filet mignon, rib eye, sirloin, skirt)
- Bison steaks
- Chicken thighs (bone-in and boneless)
- Chicken wings
- Ground beef
- Ground bison
- Ground chicken
- Ground lamb
- Ground pork
- Hot dogs (look for pure beef or beef and pork hot dogs without added sugars or other undesirable ingredients; we love high-quality beef hot dogs from Teton Waters Ranch, often sold at Costco)
- Lamb chops
- Organ meats (beef heart, beef liver)
- Pork belly
- Pork chops
- Pork roasts (butt/shoulder)
- Prosciutto
- Rack of lamb
- Salami (watch for sugars in the ingredients)
- Sausage (breakfast, Italian). Be aware of ingredients when shopping for sausage. Most brands contain corn syrup, which I stay away from. Pederson's brand has a bulk breakfast sausage that uses raw sugar and a spicy one that is sugar free. Note that the amount of sugar is so minimal that, to me, it doesn't taste sweet or cause cravings, and it doesn't even show up on the nutrition facts as a significant amount of sugar or carbs.
- Wild game

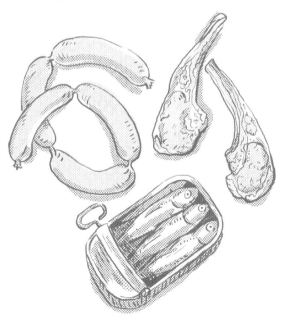

seafood

- Anchovies
- Canned cod livers
- Canned salmon
- Canned sardines
- Canned tuna
- Crab
- Lobster
- Mackerel
- Oysters (fresh or canned)
- Salmon fillets (frozen)
- Sardines
- Scallops (frozen)
- Shrimp (frozen)
- Tuna steaks

animal fats

When choosing fats for cooking, make sure to take into account the heat level you'll be using. You don't want to exceed the fat's smoke point, which is the point at which it will start to burn. I've included the smoke point for each of the recommended animal fats listed below.

- Bacon grease, collected from cooking (370°F smoke point)

- Beef suet (400°F smoke point)

- Butter (I always buy salted butter, but get what you like; if you use unsalted butter, you just might need to add a touch more salt than the recipe calls for.) (350°F smoke point)

- Duck fat (370°F smoke point)

- Ghee (485°F smoke point)

- Lard (370°F smoke point)

- Tallow (420°F smoke point)

Note:

If you're following the Lion Diet, the only fats from this list you would use are beef suet and tallow, which is rendered from beef or sheep. If you avoid dairy, you may find that you can tolerate butter because it is low in lactose; ghee, a form of clarified butter, has had the milk solids removed and therefore contains no lactose, making it a potentially even better choice. Or simply use one of the nondairy animal fats listed above.

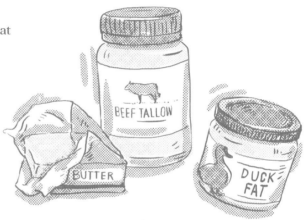

animal products (dairy and eggs)

Dairy products should be full-fat (such as whole milk, not 2% or skim) for better flavor and to hit your macro goals, and ideally raw (not pasteurized). Raw dairy tends to be gentler on the stomach and better tolerated than pasteurized. Pasteurization kills the healthy bacteria and diminishes the nutrient content.

Butter and ghee are, of course, animal products but are included in the Animal Fats list according to how they're used in cooking.

Finally, be aware that most dairy products contain carbohydrates, so keep that in mind if you're tracking your carb intake.

- Cheeses

- Cottage cheese

- Cream cheese

- Eggs (large)

- Gelatin, unflavored powdered (I use Knox unflavored gelatin, or "Gelatine." Each ¼-ounce envelope contains about 2¼ teaspoons of gelatin.)

- Heavy cream

- Kefir

- Milk

- Plain yogurt

- Sour cream

supplements

While some people do not need supplements, others feel better when supplements are added. These are some of my favorites. If you're eating plenty of fatty and bone-in meats, you're going to be getting adequate protein and collagen; however, some people struggle to eat enough, and if you're one of them, collagen peptides and protein powders may come in handy. Sometimes it's easier to drink a shake than eat a steak! People have seen great success when using colostrum for gut health and allergies. I also like to think of organ capsules as the ultimate multivitamin.

- Collagen peptides
- Colostrum
- Desiccated beef organ capsules
- Electrolyte drinks
- Protein powder (from beef, not whey)

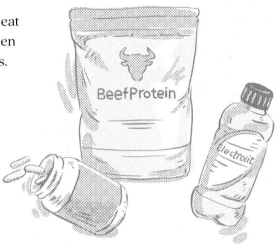

other

- Bone broth (see my recipe for homemade on page 126; store-bought broth contains herbs and spices and some brands contain sugar, so check labels)

- Cheese crackers (such as Whisps or Moon Cheese)

- Dried egg white powder

- Electrolytes (such as Beam Minerals or LMNT)

- Kosher salt (You can use any brand of this coarse salt that you like. For its purity, I prefer Redmond Real Salt's Ancient Kosher Sea Salt.)

- Meat chips (such as Carnivore Snax)

- Meat sticks (such as Chomps)

- Pork panko (You can make your own grinding up pork rinds, but I use it so often that it's convenient to purchase preground—I buy it on Amazon.)

- Pork rinds (Look for ones fried in lard and seasoned with salt. Be aware of those using vegetable oils or other seasonings. Epic, Pork King Good, and 4505 are great brands to try. Grocery store brands can also be good choices; just check the labels.)

To access discount codes for some of the products listed here, visit the "shop" section of my site (https://courtneyluna.com/shop).

kitchen tools
and small appliances

I try to keep my recipes fairly straightforward, using basic tools and equipment. Nonetheless, I do use a handful of popular small appliances to make cooking easy and quicker, in particular the air fryer and Instant Pot. Whenever possible, I give multiple cooking methods so that you can still make the recipe. Here are the items I suggest you have on hand.

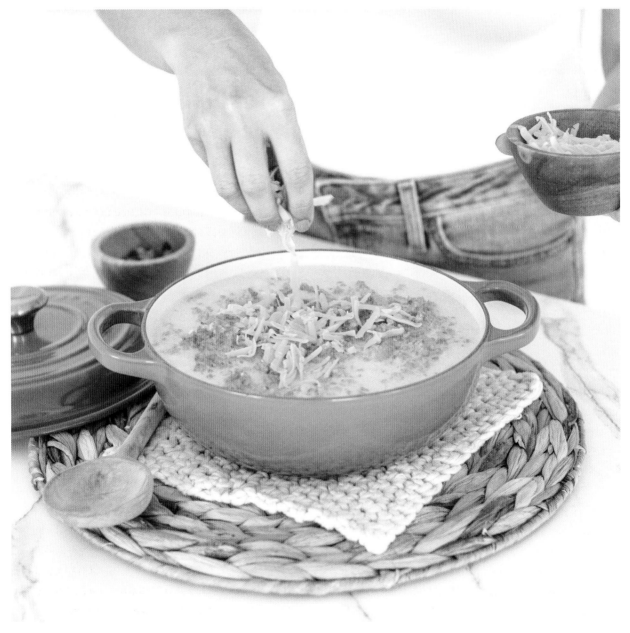

appliances

AIR FRYER: I was initially resistant to getting an air fryer (or an Instant Pot, for that matter) because I didn't want to add another appliance to my kitchen. But using the air fryer has made me a convert. It's a super convenient alternative to an oven, and it makes meat crispy. Instead of pan-searing skin-on chicken thighs on the stovetop and finishing them in the oven, you can prepare them in the air fryer and get a super crunchy skin while cooking the meat at the same time. You can think of it as using your oven, only it's quicker. I suggest you preheat your air fryer for a few minutes before using it. Some people don't like to use a microwave, so using an air fryer to rewarm foods is a great option, and it will crisp up foods such as pizza crusts and chicken skin, unlike a microwave.

BLENDER: Indispensable for recipes like Egg Bites (page 58) and Crepe Cake (page 196). If you want to make chicken flour (see my recipe on page 98), you'll need a high-powered blender; a regular blender is not sufficient. An immersion (or stick) blender is handy for making sauces like Hollandaise (page 208) and blended soups.

FOOD DEHYDRATOR: For homemade meat chips (see page 108). I recommend getting a dehydrator that has metal racks, not plastic ones. The more shelves, the better, too! You can also make jerky and even dehydrate fruit for your kids or yourself, if you're animal based.

FOOD PROCESSOR: For Dutch Baby Soufflé (page 76), Cornbread Muffins (page 90), and Meatza (page 184). For the recipes in this book, you'll need a food processor with a capacity of at least 8 cups. You'll also need a mini food processor for making dressings, sauces, and dips; mine has a 2-cup capacity.

ICE CREAM MAKER: For Carnivore Ice Cream (page 194).

INSTANT POT: I love using the Instant Pot to speed up the process of cooking tough meats. It's also fabulous for cooking eggs "hard boiled" style because when they steam, they are easier to peel. It's handy for frozen meats, too. You wouldn't want to cook frozen meat in a slow cooker because the meat might stay in the "danger zone" temperature range (between 40°F and 140°F) for too long, so the Instant Pot is perfect for last-minute meals if you forget to thaw something. This appliance has replaced my slow cooker for time and convenience. Please note that the cook times listed do not include the time it takes the Instant Pot to come to temperature or to release pressure. The time it takes to heat up depends on the quantity of liquid and food being cooked. Eggs will come to temperature quickly, while bone broth may take a while. At the end of cooking, I generally call for allowing all of the pressure to release naturally. Depending on the recipe, this can take 10 to 20 minutes.

MINI WAFFLE MAKER, NONSTICK: For All-Purpose Waffles (page 86).

SLOW COOKER, 6 TO 7 QUARTS: This appliance can be used to make Sipping Bone Broth (page 126) and Carnitas (page 160). If you have an Instant Pot, you can use it to make these recipes instead.

STAND MIXER (OPTIONAL): A great tool for hands-off mixing. It's particularly useful in the recipes for Cheesecake Mousse (page 200) and Vanilla Cupcakes with Whipped Cream Frosting (page 202). If you don't have one, a handheld electric mixer will also work.

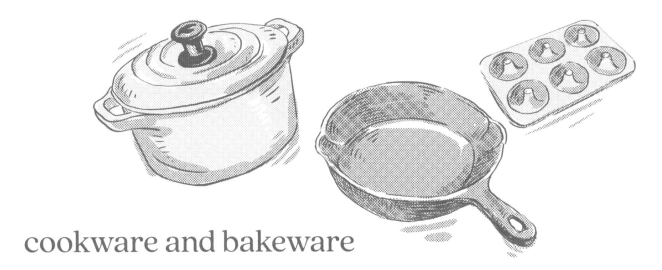

cookware and bakeware

BAKING PANS: 8-inch square baking pan, 9-inch cake pan, 9 by 5-inch loaf pan.

CASSEROLE DISHES: 13 by 9 inches and 11 by 7 inches.

CAST-IRON OR HEAVY-BOTTOMED STAINLESS-STEEL PANS: I've used cast-iron pans exclusively for the last ten years, and I love them. Nonstick cookware is not ideal because of the chemical coating used on it, and because it can't be used in the oven. Cast iron and stainless steel are better options, particularly cast iron! There's no better pan for getting a good sear on meat. For the recipes in this book, you'll need small (7- or 8-inch), medium-size (9- or 10-inch), and large (11- or 12-inch) skillets.

DONUT/MINI BAGEL PAN, SILICONE WITH 6 CAVITIES: For Mini Bagels (page 74).

DUTCH OVEN, ENAMELED, OR OTHER HEAVY SOUP POT (6 OR 7 QUARTS): For frying foods as well as making soups and pot roast.

EGG BITE MOLD: 7-well silicone mold with trivet fitted for Instant Pot.

MUFFIN PANS: Look for a standard-size 12-well metal pan with a nonstick surface for easy removal as well as a standard-size 12-well silicone muffin pan. You'll also want a nonstick 24-well mini muffin pan for making Salami Cups (page 112).

SAUCEPANS: I use these just occasionally in my cooking. The sizes used are small (2 to 4 cups) and medium (4 to 8 cups).

SHEET PANS: It's good to have at least two of these highly useful pans. I use the most common size, known as a half sheet pan, measuring 18 by 13 by 1 inch.

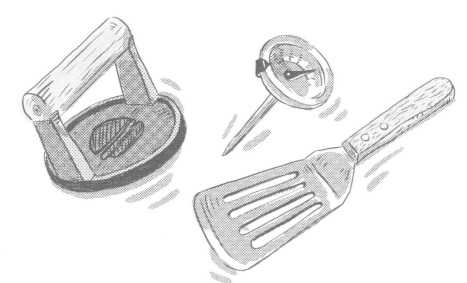

tools

BURGER SMASHER/PRESS: For 6-inch Tortillas (page 88) as well as burgers. To make larger (7- to 8-inch) tortillas, you'll need a waffle cone iron.

DEEP FRY THERMOMETER: For gauging the temperature of the tallow in the Mozzarella Sticks recipe (page 116).

KITCHEN SCALE: For best results, I suggest you weigh pork panko for baking recipes.

KNIVES: I typically use a chef's knife and a paring knife. Two of my favorite brands are Global and Wüsthof.

MEAT SLICER, ELECTRIC: For homemade meat chips (see page 108). You can also use a meat slicer to make your own deli meat and cut strips of meat for jerky. I recommend getting the most powerful slicer your budget allows—the higher the wattage, the more powerful the slicer. My meat slicer has a wattage of 200. Some also have a safety lock that must be unlocked before the machine can be turned on, which is reassuring if you have little kids.

MEAT THERMOMETER: Useful for confirming that poultry and pork are sufficiently cooked and that you don't overcook steak.

PARCHMENT PAPER SHEETS OR SILICONE MATS: I use reusable silicone mats to save on waste. These mats and parchment paper work equally well in the recipes.

SILICONE MIXING SPOONS/SPATULAS: For stirring and scraping batters, sauces, and the like.

SPATULAS, METAL AND OFFSET: For Panko Noodles (page 92).

TONGS: For turning meats and other foods.

WAFFLE CONE IRON: For 7- to 8-inch Tortillas (page 88). Waffle cone irons typically range from 7 to 8 inches in diameter (mine is 7½ inches).

WHISK: 8 to 10 inches.

WOODEN MIXING SPOONS: 12 inches.

how to use *the* recipes

By nature, carnivore cooking is fairly straightforward, using a limited number of ingredients and a range of cooking techniques best suited to meat (you will not, for example, be using a steaming basket to make the recipes in this book!). But before jumping in, please take a moment to read my recipe tips to ensure your success in the kitchen.

icons

To quickly find recipes that use an air fryer, Instant Pot, or slow cooker, look for handy icons at the top of the page.

serving sizes

The portion sizes in this book are based on the average person eating roughly 1½ pounds of boneless meat or up to 3 pounds of bone-in meat per day, with each serving being ½ pound of boneless meat or ¾ to 1 pound of bone-in meat. If a recipe is enriched with eggs or dairy, the amount of meat needed per person is generally slightly less. If the meat is served with another food, like carnivore noodles, that also may stretch the amount of meat needed per person. Note that since everyone's hunger levels and macronutrient needs are unique, you may find yourself needing more or less food per day. Feel free to adjust the portion sizes to suit your specific needs.

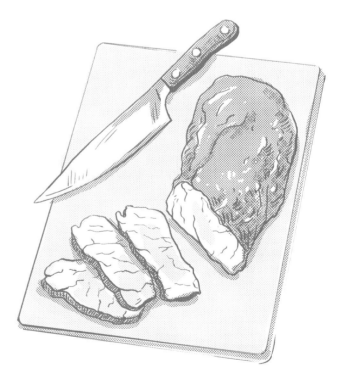

seasonings

Let's address the elephant in the room. You might look at some of the recipes in this book and think, "Where are the seasonings?" Just so you know, you're not alone; half of the internet asks me that same question.

For starters, seasonings other than salt are not strict carnivore because they come from plants. But, like coffee and tea, they get a free pass. If you tolerate seasonings and using them helps you stick to this way of eating, then go for it. I find that most carnivores do not use spices, though. Once you've adapted, the flavor of meat seasoned with a high-quality salt is enough. Just like an ex-smoker might say their taste buds came alive after they quit smoking, the same goes for what you eat. My preferences changed after I went carnivore; garlic and onions taste super strong to me now, and I prefer most of my meat simply salted. Smoked salt is a great option for extra flavor. I do get a little wild with some cinnamon and vanilla extract in my desserts, but know that all of these additions are optional.

If you're coming to carnivore to address autoimmune issues, I would omit all seasonings other than salt in the beginning and then try adding them back in later.

Feel free to add your favorite seasonings to any of the recipes in this book; they're here to be a guide for you, and you are more than welcome to make them your own.

cooking with animal fats

There are many different animal fats you can experiment with; see page 26 for ideas. In my cooking, I keep it simple, using just three: tallow, bacon grease, and butter. (*Note:* If you are following the lion diet, you should use only tallow and/or beef suet.)

Tallow is an ideal all-purpose cooking fat: it is fairly neutral-tasting and has a high smoke point (420°F), so you can use it for any preparation, from sautéing to deep-frying. Rendered bacon grease is another great choice because it is cost-effective—you save the grease that is released when you cook bacon—and it adds a rich taste. (Note that the smoke point of bacon grease is lower than tallow, at 370°F.) Butter adds a nice flavor, too, but its smoke point is even lower (350°F), so while it works well for cooking eggs, it can burn if cooked high and long. If you want to use butter for cooking a steak, I recommend you pair it with an equal amount of tallow to keep the butter from burning, or add the butter at the end of cooking. Another buttery option is ghee, which has a smoke point of 485°F, but is expensive.

When a recipe gives you the choice of using another heat-tolerant fat in place of tallow, feel free to use any fat you like from the list on page 26, other than butter.

cooking with parmesan cheese

Many of my recipes call for shredded Parmesan cheese. I use the preshredded type sold in bags or tubs. The one I purchase is aged for ten months, which makes the Parmesan less dry and more versatile than traditional Parmigiano-Reggiano from Italy, which is aged for at least two years. However, in the recipe for Creamy Chicken Casserole with Crunchy Panko Topping (page 170), I use the much drier pregrated Parmesan, the kind that is sold in a can and is shelf-stable. This type of Parmesan is required to give that dish its crispy topping.

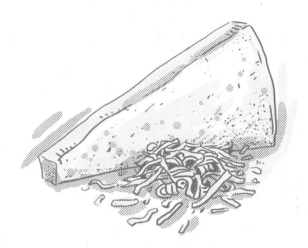

meat cooking techniques

You will use many different meat cooking methods for the recipes in this book. Here is a list of the key techniques:

- **SEARING:** Great for quick-cooking cuts, like steaks. To ensure even cooking, thicker steaks are seared to create a nice crust and then finished in the oven. My top-secret searing tip: After searing the first side of a piece of meat, flip the meat over onto a not-yet-used part of the skillet. This will enhance browning since that area of the skillet surface will be hotter.

- **BRAISING:** This method uses both a quick sear and a slow simmer in a liquid in the oven, such as when making a pot roast. The liquid normally comes about halfway up the side of the meat.

- **PAN-FRYING:** For quickly cooking foods such as ground meat, cubed steak, meatballs, and patties.

- **BAKING:** Using indirect dry heat is great for finishing off a seared filet or baking carnivore bread or muffins.

- **BROILING:** Using direct heat from above, broiling is often employed to brown or crisp the top of a dish such as a casserole or to get the ends of a piece of meat crispy (as in my Carnitas recipe on page 160).

- **PRESSURE COOKING:** This quick cooking technique works well for tough cuts of meat, such as brisket. It also allows you to cook meats safely from frozen. The Instant Pot is a popular appliance for pressure cooking.

food storage guidelines

Generally, prepared foods can be kept in the refrigerator for up to five days and may be frozen for up to six months. Exceptions to this rule are noted in the recipes.

Anything made with eggs—including breads, muffins, tortillas, and noodles—should be stored in the refrigerator, not on the counter.

Saturated fats, such as butter, tallow, and bacon grease, can be stored at room temperature. I keep backup butter in the fridge, but always have a stick on the counter for cooking. Butter can also be frozen.

If freezing items stacked one atop the other, like hamburger patties or tortillas, be sure to slip a sheet of parchment paper between them so that you can easily separate them once frozen and remove just the amount you need.

In my freezer, you will always find a variety of cuts of beef, labeled and dated, ready to be pulled out, thawed, and cooked. As I mentioned in the "Shopping Tips" sidebar on page 24, it is very economical to buy a portion of a cow from a local farmer. I get a quarter cow to have my own personal stash of meat on hand. I also keep all my seafood frozen: salmon, red Argentine shrimp, and scallops. Portions can easily be thawed the night before you plan to cook them.

reheating guidelines

Many prepared foods can be reheated equally well in a preheated moderate oven (350°F), air fryer, toaster oven, or microwave. However, if the food has a crispy or crusty exterior, an oven, air fryer, or toaster oven should be used to maintain the desired texture.

If the prepared food is moist, like a stew or pot roast, and you want to avoid drying it out, then the microwave or a covered pot on the stovetop over medium heat is the best choice.

Egg dishes can be reheated in the microwave, but briefly, just until warmed, and ideally using low or moderate power; too much time in the microwave will cause eggs to become rubbery. I suggest you reheat eggs in thirty-second increments.

Likewise, sauces made with cream and/or cheese should be reheated gently either in the microwave or in a saucepan on the stovetop. Overheating dairy products when reheating them can cause them to break or curdle.

Noodles can be rewarmed in the microwave.

For steaks, a quick warm-up in the air fryer or in a hot skillet is best to keep a nice crust on the outside. After searing, you could cover the pan with a lid, creating a sort of oven to warm up the center of the steak.

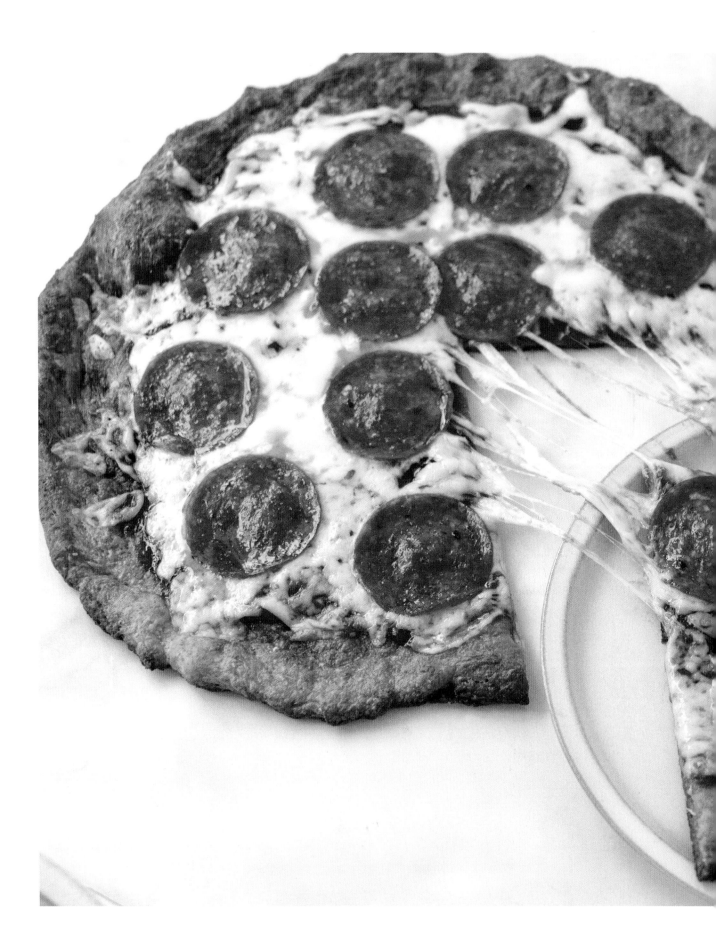

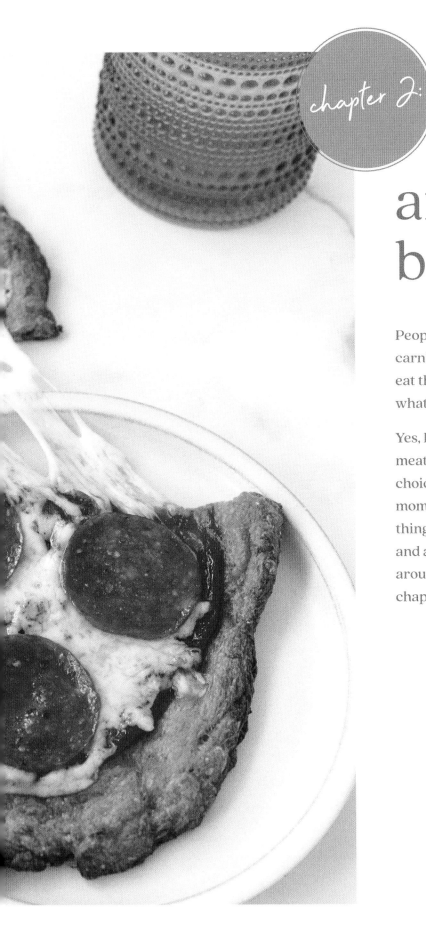

animal-based kids

People ask me all the time if my kids eat a carnivore diet, too. Because children should eat their fruits and vegetables, right? That's what we've all been told again and again!

Yes, I feed my children a diet that is mostly meat, and I feel 100 percent confident in this choice. However, I'm also a busy working mom, so I've found some ways to make things a little easier on myself as a parent, and a little easier on my kids when they're around their peers. That's what this short chapter is all about.

animal based *versus* carnivore

We take an animal-based approach with our kids because it makes things a little more sustainable for them. As explained in Chapter 1, animal based is carnivore (meat plus animal products like eggs and dairy) with the addition of fruit, honey, and maple syrup. The reason fruit is included, rather than vegetables, is because the fruit is the least toxic part of a plant. Our kids eat everything we eat with the addition of some fruit and the occasional slice of sourdough bread (if eating traditional bread, sourdough is the best option since it's better on the gut than other types of breads).

Here is what an example of a day of eating looks like for them:

breakfast: bacon, steak, and eggs

snack: a couple of strawberries and a string cheese

lunch: cheeseburger patties

snack: full-fat Greek yogurt with no-sugar-added jam or a protein shake (see sidebar)

dinner: a creative recipe like Carnizza (page 182) or "Corn" Dogs (page 188)

bedtime snack: a banana and a glass of whole (preferably raw) milk

Let's be honest, I could probably add a few more snacks in there. Even though my kids eat nutrient-dense meals, they like to snack, as all children do. I just try to make their snacks look like mini meals so they're eating a healthy balance of protein and fat.

MY KIDS' FAVORITE PROTEIN SHAKE

My kids have an animal-based protein shake almost every day. In fact, they are obsessed with it! I do a blend of raw milk, a splash of heavy cream, strawberry-flavored beef protein powder, a scoop of colostrum, the contents of a desiccated organ supplement capsule, and a handful of frozen fruit. If you don't have access to raw milk, you can use organic whole milk, preferably A2 if you can't find raw, because it is easier on digestion.

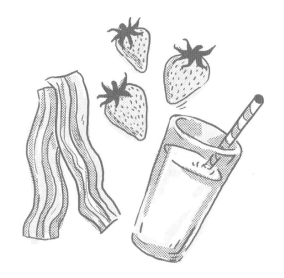

making room
for treats *and* choices

Educating our kids on nutrition is the most important thing we do. I don't want to demonize food, but rather help them be aware of what food does to their bodies and how they feel after eating. I don't want them to feel deprived and go to a friend's house and binge on all the things Mom won't let them have. That is why part of our approach as parents is to occasionally give them control over the food choices they make. If we go to a birthday party, for example, we will feed them a healthy animal-based meal beforehand, and then, while we're at the party, they're allowed to eat what they want, within reason. If they want cake, we just remind them that they do not need to eat the whole piece, to listen to their body and pay attention to how it makes them feel. Later, when they're running around like banshees, we gently bring up how they're acting, ask them how their tummies are, and remind them that eating those types of foods can make us not feel our best.

Everything we have in the house is food that I can say yes to. For breakfast, I give the kids some suggestions and let them pick what they want from that list. I feel like a line cook at Denny's sometimes, but this allows them to feel like they're in control, and who doesn't want a say in what they eat? As adults, we have that choice for every meal, so I feel it's important to offer it to children as well. However, dinner is whatever I serve, and I tell them they can go to bed hungry if they don't like it (ha!). But I do make sure to offer something I know they like. If I'm trying a new recipe, I make sure to provide a "safe" food for them that I know they'll eat. On the correct colored plate, of course—oh, toddlers...

On the rare occasion the kids have a treat, it's outside of the home; that way, there aren't leftovers of said treat that they are constantly asking for. I also limit the amount of fruit they have, because even though the sugar is from a "healthy" source, it still affects their behavior and makes them wild. And when they do eat fruit, we teach them to pair it with a protein to help keep their blood sugar stable. Some examples of pairings are berries and a cheese stick, or dried mango with salami and/or cheese slices. Fruit is served with a meal, as opposed to putting it on a pedestal as a treat for finishing their protein.

Focusing on prioritizing meats and animal products and paying attention to macros (like pairing their fruit with protein) seems to be working well in teaching my children how to nourish their bodies. While they do love simple meals like bacon, steak, and eggs, we have fun with my recipes to keep this way of eating exciting, creative, and sustainable for them.

family meals

There's no rule that you can't have a traditional dinner recipe for breakfast, but we usually serve steak, bacon, sausage, eggs, yogurt, and some fruit. On the weekend, Mini Bagels (page 74) or Cinnamon Rolls (page 78) might make an appearance (my kids love them). Another fun and easy idea is pork rind cereal—Carnivore Crispies! Hear me out, because it tastes better than it sounds! Take some regular salted pork rinds, place them in a bowl, and break them into bite-sized chunks. Add a sprinkle of cinnamon if you'd like, and for the milk use either whole milk (it does have carbs), half-and-half, or whole milk with a drizzle of heavy cream. Pop an ice cube in there so it stays cold. Curious what this tastes like? The version without cinnamon reminds me of how Rice Krispies taste before you dump a spoonful of sugar on them. Tons of people have been surprised by how delicious pig skin cereal is, even though they were scared to try it. I'm forever grateful to my carnivore buddy, Bee, for sharing this idea; now it's one of my favorite treats.

Lunches are typically kept simple—burger patties, steaks, chicken wings, deli meat roll-ups, a charcuterie plate with fruit for the kids, or leftovers from previous dinners.

Dinner is often a creative recipe from this book.

While my kids love all of my recipes (okay, the majority of them, I should say), there are a few fan favorites:

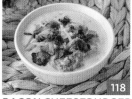
118
BACON CHEESEBURGER SOUP

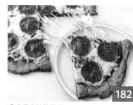
182
CARNIZZA

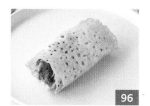
96
CHEESE WRAP

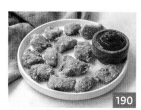
190
CHICKEN NUGGETS

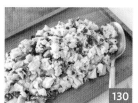
130
CHICKEN SALAD

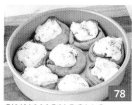
78
CINNAMON ROLLS

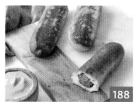
188
"CORN" DOGS

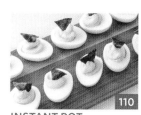
110
INSTANT POT DEVILED EGGS

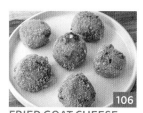
106
FRIED GOAT CHEESE BALLS

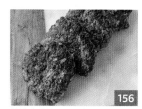
156
HIDDEN LIVER BURGERS

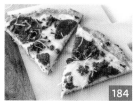
184
MEATZA

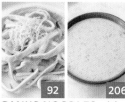
92 **206**
PANKO NOODLES with BROWNED BUTTER CREAM SAUCE

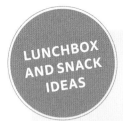

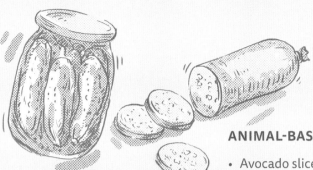

- Bacon
- Cheese crackers (made of only cheese)
- Cheese sticks (made of only cheese)
- Deli turkey + cheese roll-ups
- Hard-boiled eggs
- Meat chips (for homemade, see page 108)
- Meat sticks
- Pork rinds
- Salami

ANIMAL-BASED ADDITIONS:

- Avocado slices
- Fresh berries or other fruit
- Dried fruit without added sugar
- Natural fruit chips (freeze-dried or baked)
- Olives
- Pickles
- Salted plantain chips (preferably cooked in coconut oil)

Always check the ingredients to make sure the meat sticks, pickles, and fruit chips you buy don't have added sugar, that the pork rinds are fried in lard and not vegetable oil.

Instead of serving one protein and two side dishes for dinner like I did in our pre-carnivore days, I like to offer a couple of different animals at most meals to keep things interesting. So, if I make a single meat like brisket (page 138), I add a couple of other options, such as a plate of bacon and some grilled halloumi or similar cheese. Is your family getting tired of burgers every day? Try switching up the cuts or types of meats.

If you have picky eaters at home, get your kids involved in the shopping and cooking process. My older child loves to look at the different meats at the grocery store (especially the whole fish and chicken feet—eek!), and they both love it when I cook outside on the grill. We put on music when I'm outside cooking and they like to have a grill dance party. It's also fun to set out a huge platter of different meats and cheeses and go to town. We enjoy a family-style meal of sliced steak, bacon, burger patties, grilled cheese, and shrimp. Kids love to eat with their hands, so sometimes I even throw down some parchment paper, toss all the food on the table, and then we feast. It feels primal, too.

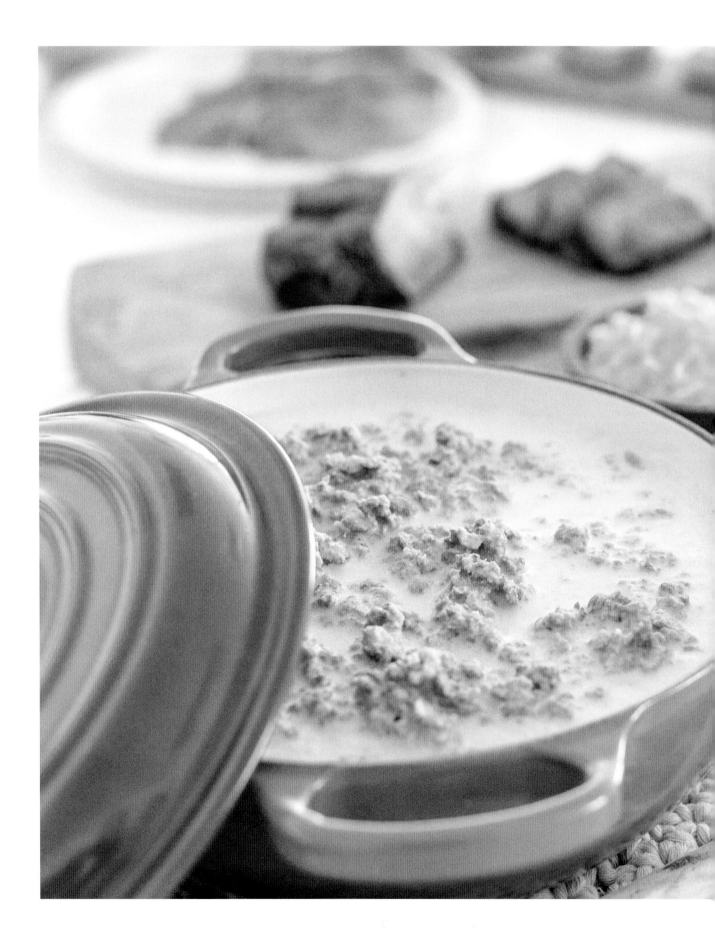

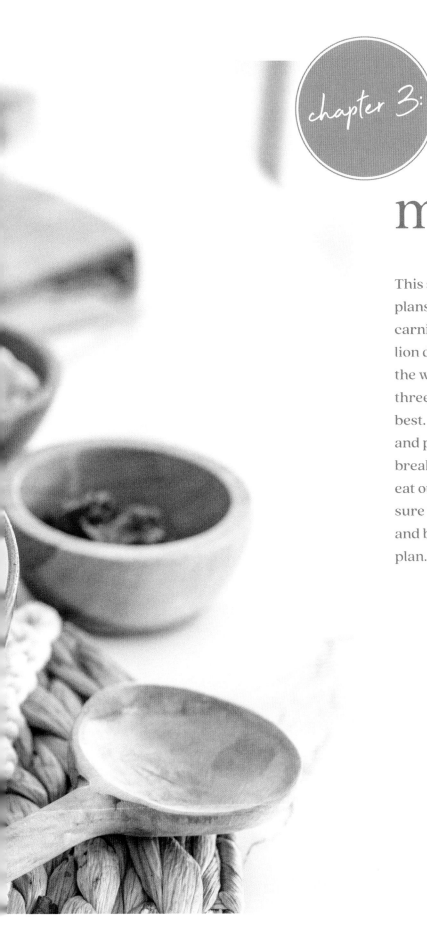

meal plans

This section features three one-week meal plans, each for a different version of the carnivore diet: standard, dairy-free, and lion diet. Choose the plan that matches the way you are currently eating, or try all three and see which one makes you feel the best. Each seven-day plan feeds two people and provides all of the meals needed for breakfast, lunch, and dinner. If you like to eat out sometimes during the week, make sure to adjust the shopping list accordingly, and be sure to order food that keeps to the plan.

Please use these plans as a guide. You may even make substitutions as you need to; just make sure they comply with the plan you are following. Generally, one serving consists of ½ pound of boneless meat; however, if a dish is enriched with eggs and/or dairy, the amount of meat per serving tends to be less. That said, keep in mind that everyone's macronutrient and caloric goals are different—based on gender, age, and physical activity—and that a serving size for you might be larger or smaller than a serving size for somebody else. If you have leftovers, simply freeze them for later, to be enjoyed after you've completed the meal plan you are following.

Recipes that need to be doubled for the plan are labeled "x2." Some are doubled to make enough for two servings, and some to create leftovers for another meal later in the week, keeping you from having to cook every meal from scratch. See page 35 for general storage and reheating guidelines for prepared foods. For any recipe that calls for egg yolks or whites alone, save the leftover whites or yolks for use in another recipe to avoid wasting good food. Note that when the amount of bacon to be used in a recipe is given in number of slices, I've specified regular, thin-cut bacon for accurate portioning since that is the type I use. If you prefer thick-cut bacon, that's fine—simply cut the number of slices used by one-third or one-half, depending on the thickness of your bacon.

Finally, the grocery lists that follow the plans do not include any of the seasonings and ingredients marked as optional in the recipes, so if you plan to include those, make sure you have the additional ingredients you need on hand or add them down to the shopping list.

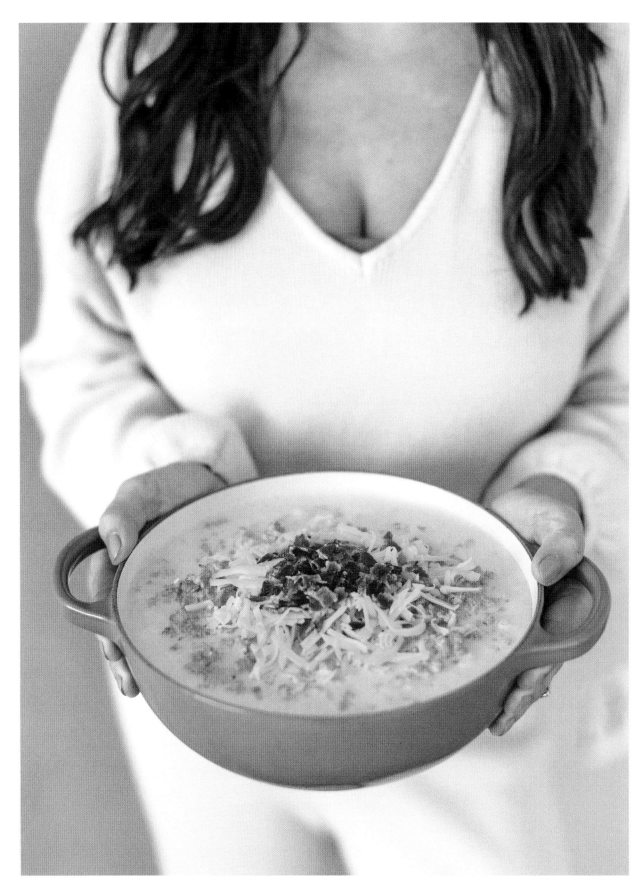

standard carnivore
meal plan

	BREAKFAST	LUNCH	DINNER	*Notes:*

Sunday:

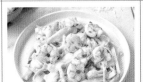

BISCUITS AND GRAVY* `72`

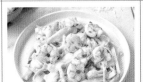

AIR FRYER SHRIMP and 4 slices cooked regular, thin-cut bacon** `142`

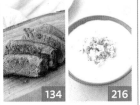

FILET MIGNON with BLUE CHEESE CREAM SAUCE *** `134` `216`

*Make a half batch of English Muffins to be used for this meal and later in the week. For this meal, you'll use one-quarter of the gravy (about ¾ cup) and 1 English muffin for each serving (or 1½ cups gravy and 2 muffins total). Store 2 of the remaining muffins and the gravy in the refrigerator for breakfast on Tuesday; freeze the remaining 2 muffins for breakfast on Saturday.

**You will use a total of 26 slices (about 1½ pounds) of regular, thin-cut bacon for several meals through Wednesday. I suggest you batch-cook this quantity. For an easier, hands-off method, try my method for baking bacon on page 166. Be sure to reserve the bacon grease for cooking later in the week.

***For this meal, you will use about ¼ cup of the sauce for each serving (or about ½ cup total). You will use the remaining sauce for dinner on Thursday.

Monday:

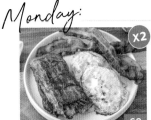

`x2`

BREAKFAST OF CHAMPIONS using leftover bacon `60`

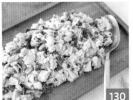

CHICKEN SALAD, using leftover bacon* `130`

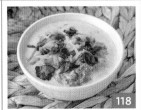

BACON CHEESEBURGER SOUP** using leftover bacon `118`

*Save the leftover egg whites from making Butter Bacon Mayo for the noodles called for in tomorrow's lunch of Ramen.

**For this meal, you'll be using the entire batch of soup, divided into 2 servings.

Tuesday:

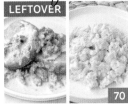

`LEFTOVER`

BISCUITS AND GRAVY and COTTAGE CHEESE EGGS `70`

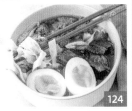

RAMEN using leftover bacon `124`

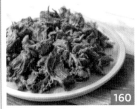

CARNITAS* `160`

*For this meal, you will use 2 servings of the Carnitas. Set aside 1 ⅓ cups for lunch on Thursday. Freeze the remaining portion for later, to be enjoyed after you've completed the meal plan. Note that Carnitas is also used in the Dairy-Free Carnivore Meal Plan.

	BREAKFAST	LUNCH	DINNER	*Notes:*

Wednesday:

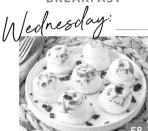
58

INSTANT POT BACON AND GRUYÈRE EGG BITES using leftover bacon

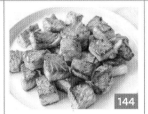
144

SALMON BITES

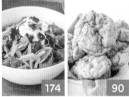
174 | 90

CHILI and CORNBREAD MUFFINS*

*You will use 2 servings of chili and 2 cornbread muffins for this meal and another 2 servings of chili with 2 muffins for lunch on Saturday. Freeze the remaining 2 servings of chili and remaining 4 muffins for later.

Thursday:

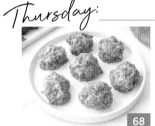
68

BREAKFAST MEATBALLS*

LEFTOVER

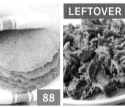
88

4 soft tacos made with 6-inch **TORTILLAS**, filled with 1 ⅓ cups leftover **CARNITAS**, ½ cup shredded cheddar cheese (about 2 ounces), and ¼ cup sour cream**

LEFTOVER

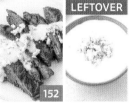
152

½ batch **PAN-SEARED SKIRT STEAK** with leftover **BLUE CHEESE CREAM SAUCE**

*For this meal, you'll be serving 4 meatballs per person, or 8 total. Freeze the remaining meatballs for later.

**The tortilla recipe yields eight 6-inch tortillas, twice as many as you need for this meal. You can freeze the 4 leftover tortillas for later. To have just enough tortillas for this meal, make a half batch of tortillas, adjusting the amounts of ingredients accordingly.

Friday:

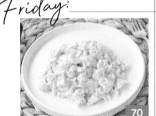
70

COTTAGE CHEESE EGGS, add 4 slices cooked regular, thin-cut bacon*

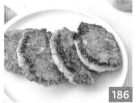
186

TUNA MELT PATTIES

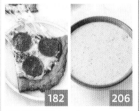
182 | 206

CARNIZZA using ½ batch **BROWNED BUTTER CREAM SAUCE** and 1 to 2 ounces pepperoni slices or leftover cooked meat for topping**

*You will use 8 slices (about ½ pound) of cooked regular, thin-cut bacon for breakfast today and tomorrow. I suggest you batch-cook this quantity. For an easier, hands-off method, try my method for baking bacon on page 166.

**For this meal, you'll consume the entire pizza, or ½ pizza per person. A half batch of the cream sauce may be more than you need to top the pizza; reserve any leftovers for after you've completed the plan.

Saturday:

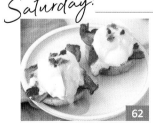
62

½ batch **EGGS BENEDICT** using leftover **ENGLISH MUFFINS** and leftover bacon, but make a full batch of **HOLLANDAISE SAUCE***

LEFTOVER | LEFTOVER

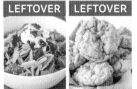

CHILI and CORNBREAD MUFFINS

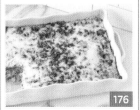
176

WHITE LASAGNA**

*The hollandaise sauce cannot be made in a half batch for this meal, but leftovers can be kept for up to 4 days and be rewarmed.

**You will be using 2 servings of lasagna for the meal plan. Enjoy the remaining servings next week, or freeze for later.

dairy-free carnivore
meal plan

Because butter is low in lactose, some dairy-free carnivores include it in their diet. If you do not tolerate it, for any recipe calling for butter, you may swap it for tallow or another animal fat.

BREAKFAST	LUNCH	DINNER	*Notes:*

Sunday:

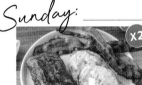 **x2** `60`

BREAKFAST OF CHAMPIONS*

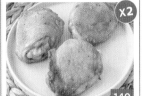 **x2** `140`

CRISPY CHICKEN THIGHS**

 `174` `90`

CHILI (omit cheese and sour cream toppings) and CORNBREAD MUFFINS***

**A double batch makes 4 servings. Reserve the remaining 2 servings for lunch on Thursday.

***You will use 2 servings of chili and 2 muffins for this meal and another 2 servings of chili with 2 muffins for lunch on Tuesday. Freeze the remaining 2 servings of chili and remaining 4 muffins for later.

*You will use a total of 24 slices (about 1 ⅓ pounds) of cooked regular, thin-cut bacon for several meals through Thursday. I suggest you batch-cook this quantity. For an easier, hands-off method, try my method for baking bacon on page 166. Be sure to reserve the bacon grease for cooking later in the week

Monday:

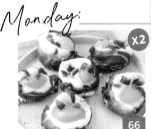 **x2** `66`

PROSCIUTTO EGG CUPS (omit cheese)*

*For this meal, you will be serving 3 egg cups per person, or 6 total. Save the remaining egg cups for breakfast on Wednesday.

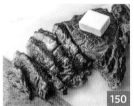 `150`

PAN-SEARED RIB EYE

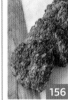 `156` `86`

2 HIDDEN LIVER BURGERS topped with 4 slices leftover bacon, served on 4 **ALL-PURPOSE WAFFLES****

**For this meal, you'll make a half batch of the burgers, omitting the egg. One batch of waffles will give you more than you need; freeze the remainder for later. Mini waffle makers vary in size; if the waffle recipe makes 8 waffles using your mini waffle maker, make a half batch for this meal, adjusting the quantity of ingredients needed accordingly.

Tuesday:

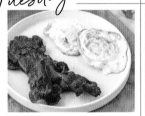

4 eggs over-easy (see page 60 for my frying method) and 4 slices leftover bacon

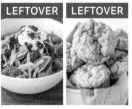 **LEFTOVER** **LEFTOVER**

CHILI and CORNBREAD MUFFINS

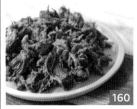 `160`

CARNITAS*

*Freeze the leftover Carnitas for after you've completed this meal plan. Note that Carnitas is also used in the Standard Carnivore Meal Plan.

BREAKFAST	LUNCH	DINNER	*Notes:*

Wednesday:

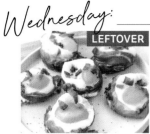
LEFTOVER

PROSCIUTTO EGG CUPS

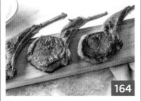
164

LAMB LOLLIPOPS

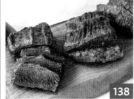
138

INSTANT POT SMOKED BRISKET*

*For this meal, you'll be using about one-third of the brisket, divided into 2 servings, or one-sixth per person. Freeze the leftover brisket for after you've completed this meal plan. (Note that smoked brisket is used for a couple of meals in the Lion Diet meal plan.)

Thursday:

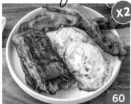
x2
60

BREAKFAST OF CHAMPIONS using leftover bacon

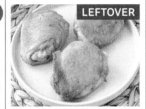
LEFTOVER

CRISPY CHICKEN THIGHS

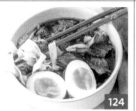
124

RAMEN using leftover bacon

Friday:

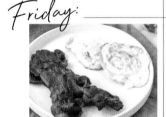

4 eggs over-easy (see method, page 60) and 4 slices cooked regular, thin-cut bacon

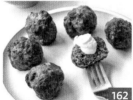
162

KOFTA MEATBALLS (omit feta dip)*

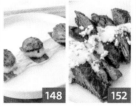
148   152

½ batch PAN-SEARED SCALLOPS and PAN-SEARED SKIRT STEAK**

*This recipe makes double what you need for the meal plan. Enjoy leftovers by the middle of next week, or freeze for later.

**Set aside 2 servings of steak for breakfast tomorrow morning. If you find ½ pound of steak along with ¼ pound of scallops to be too much food for this meal, freeze any leftover steak for later.

Saturday:

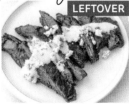
LEFTOVER

PAN-SEARED SKIRT STEAK with 4 poached eggs (see page 62 for my poaching method)

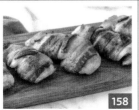
158

BACON-WRAPPED CHICKEN THIGHS*

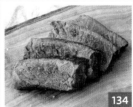
134

FILET MIGNON

*You will have 1 extra serving. Enjoy the leftover portion within 5 days, or freeze for later.

lion diet
meal plan

For any recipe calling for butter, swap it out for tallow and omit any optional seasonings.

	BREAKFAST	LUNCH	DINNER	Notes:
Sunday:	**150** PAN-SEARED RIB EYE	**136** POT ROAST*	**134** FILET MIGNON	*For this meal, you'll be using half of the pot roast, or one-quarter per serving. You'll eat the remainder as leftovers for dinner on Tuesday.
Monday:	**152** PAN-SEARED SKIRT STEAK*	**156** HIDDEN LIVER BURGERS (omit egg)	**138** INSTANT POT SMOKED BRISKET**	*For this meal, you'll be using one-half of the steak, or 2 servings; divide the remaining steak into 2 equal portions, freezing one for later and reserving the other for lunch on Tuesday. **For this meal, you'll be using about one-third of the smoked brisket, divided into 2 servings, or one-sixth per person. Set aside another third of the brisket for breakfast on Thursday. Freeze the remaining third for later, after you've completed this meal plan.
Tuesday:	**150** PAN-SEARED RIB EYE	LEFTOVER **154** ½ batch PAN-SEARED HEART and PAN-SEARED SKIRT STEAK*	LEFTOVER POT ROAST	*The average size of a beef heart is too large for two servings, but heart is best served freshly prepared (it doesn't reheat well). I recommend you cut the raw heart in half, cooking one half for today's meal and freezing the other half to be prepared fresh later on. Divide the single serving of leftover steak in two so that each person has ¼ pound of steak to accompany the heart.

BREAKFAST	LUNCH	DINNER	Notes:

Wednesday:

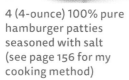

4 (4-ounce) 100% pure hamburger patties seasoned with salt (see page 156 for my cooking method)

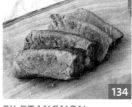
134
FILET MIGNON

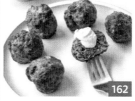
162
KOFTA MEATBALLS (omit feta dip)*

*For this meal, you'll be using half of the meatballs. You'll eat the remaining meatballs for breakfast on Friday.

Thursday:

LEFTOVER
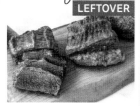
INSTANT POT SMOKED BRISKET

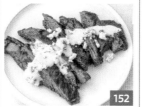
152
PAN-SEARED SKIRT STEAK*

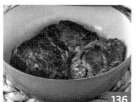
136
POT ROAST**

*You will use 2 servings of steak for this meal and the remaining 2 servings for lunch on Friday.

**For this meal, you'll be using half of the pot roast. You'll eat the remainder as leftovers for lunch on Saturday.

Friday:

LEFTOVER
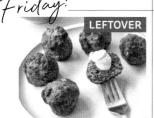
KOFTA MEATBALLS

LEFTOVER
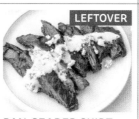
PAN-SEARED SKIRT STEAK

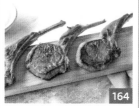
164
LAMB LOLLIPOPS

Saturday:

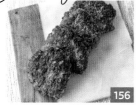
156
HIDDEN LIVER BURGERS (omit egg)

LEFTOVER
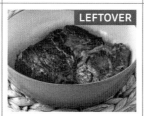
POT ROAST

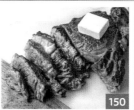
150
PAN-SEARED RIB EYE

standard carnivore
grocery list

MEATS

Bacon, thin-cut, 2 pounds

Beef, shaved, 8 ounces

Breakfast sausage, bulk, 2 pounds

Chicken breasts, boneless, skinless, 1 pound

Filet mignons, about 1½ inches thick, 2 (8 ounces)

Ground beef, 3 pounds

Ground chicken, 1 pound

Italian sausage, bulk, 1 pound

Pepperoni slices, 2 ounces (for Carnizza; omit if using leftover meat as topping)

Pork butt/shoulder, boneless, 4 pounds

Red Argentine or other jumbo shrimp, frozen, 1 pound

Salmon fillet, skinless, 1 pound

Sirloin steak, boneless, 1 pound

Skirt steak, 1¾ pounds

DAIRY AND EGGS

Blue cheese, 5 ounces

Butter, salted, 6 sticks (1½ pounds)

Cheddar cheese, shredded, 11 ounces

Cottage cheese, 4 ounces (½ cup)

Cream cheese, 3 (8-ounce) blocks

Eggs, large, 5 dozen

Gruyère cheese, 2 ounces

Heavy cream, 1 quart

Mozzarella cheese, shredded, 18 ounces

Parmesan cheese, shredded, 18 ounces

Ricotta cheese, 15-ounce container

Sour cream, 8-ounce container

PANTRY ITEMS

Beef broth, 3 cups (or, if making homemade, 3 pounds beef bones and 8 ounces marrow bones)

Chicken broth, 5 cups (or, if making homemade, 3 pounds chicken bones and 8 ounces chicken feet)

Distilled white vinegar

Gelatin, unflavored, 6 tablespoons

Lemon, 1 small

Pork panko, 16 ounces

Solid tuna in water, 5-ounce can

Tallow, ½ cup (about ⅓ [11-ounce] jar)

dairy-free carnivore
grocery list

MEATS

Bacon, thin-cut, 2 pounds

Beef brisket, 3 pounds

Beef liver, 2 ounces

Beef, shaved, 8 ounces

Chicken thighs, bone-in, skin-on, 4 pounds

Chicken thighs, boneless, skinless, 6 (about 1½ pounds)

Filet mignons, about 1½ inches thick, 2 (8 ounces)

Ground beef, 2½ pounds

Ground chicken, 1 pound

Ground lamb, 1 pound

Pork butt/shoulder, boneless, 4 pounds

Prosciutto, 12 slices (about 6 ounces)

Rack of lamb, frenched, about 1½ pounds

Rib eye steak, boneless, about 1½ inches thick, 1 (1 pound)

Sea scallops, 8 ounces

Skirt steak, 3½ pounds

Sirloin steak, boneless, 1 pound

DAIRY AND EGGS

Butter, salted, 2 sticks (8 ounces), or ¾ cup plus 2 tablespoons tallow (about ¾ [11-ounce] jar)

Eggs, large, 4½ dozen

PANTRY ITEMS

Beef broth, 2 cups (or, if making homemade, 3 pounds bones and 8 ounces marrow bones)

Chicken broth, 5 cups (or, if making homemade, 3 pounds bones and 8 ounces chicken feet)

Gelatin, unflavored, 2 tablespoons

Pork panko, 9 ounces

Tallow, 6 tablespoons plus 1 teaspoon (about ⅓ [11-ounce] jar)

lion diet
grocery list

MEATS

Beef brisket, 3 pounds

Beef heart, 1 (about 2 pounds)

Beef liver, 8 ounces

Chuck roasts, boneless, 2 (2½ pounds)

Filet mignons, about 1½ inches thick, 4 (8 ounces)

Ground beef, 4 pounds

Ground lamb, 1 pound

Rack of lamb, frenched, about 1½ pounds

Rib-eye steaks, boneless, about 1½ inches thick, 3 (1 pound)

Skirt steak, 4 pounds

PANTRY ITEMS

Beef broth, 2 cups (or, if making homemade, 3 pounds beef bones and 8 ounces marrow bones)

Tallow, 11-ounce jar

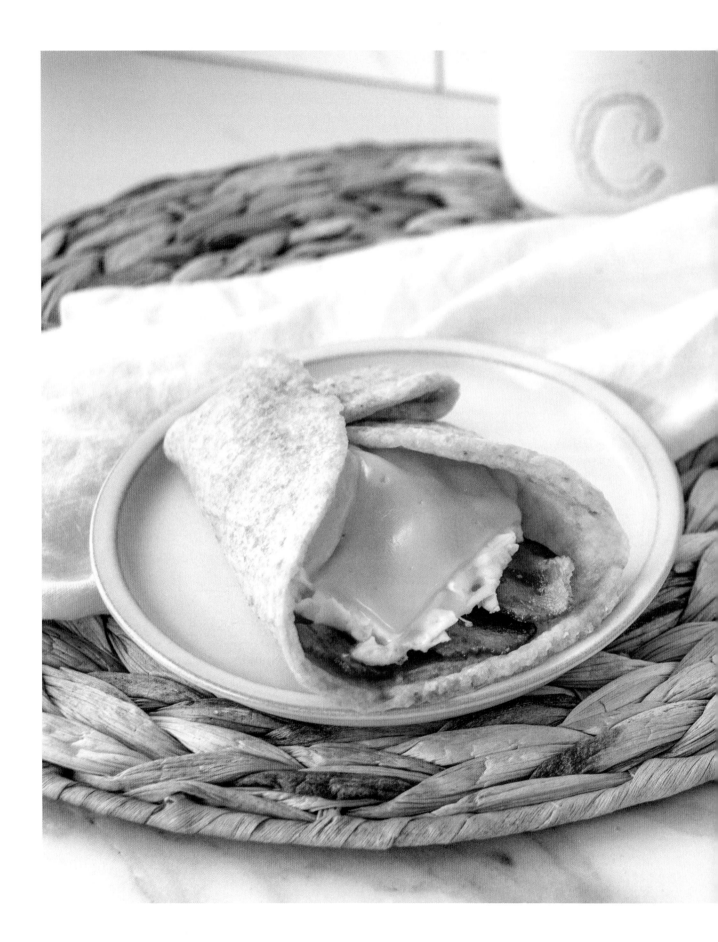

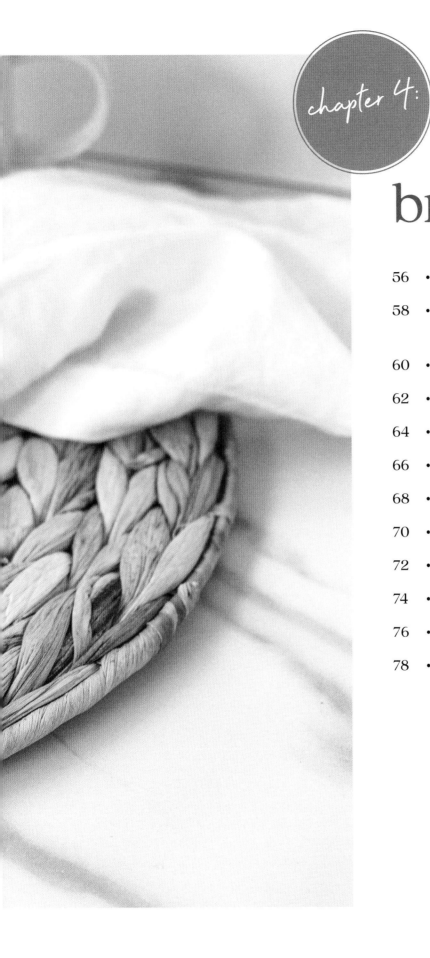

breakfast

breakfast casserole

YIELD:
8 servings

PREP TIME:
20 minutes

COOK TIME:
1 hour

I love meal prepping this casserole for the week. It's also good to have on a morning when guests are visiting—make it ahead and rewarm it, or prep the casserole the night before and bake it fresh in the morning. It's a comfy dish and makes a great base for your own creative spins. Switch up the ground meats, add some cooked bacon or a sprinkle of cheddar cheese, or go wherever your heart takes you.

1 tablespoon salted butter, for the dish

1 teaspoon bacon grease or tallow, for the pan

1 pound bulk sausage (any type)

1 pound ground beef

2½ teaspoons kosher salt, divided

12 large eggs

1 (8-ounce) package cream cheese

1 cup sour cream

1. Preheat the oven to 350°F. Grease a 13 by 9-inch casserole dish with the butter.

2. Preheat a large skillet over medium-high heat until it begins to smoke. Drop in the bacon grease and swirl to coat the pan, then add the sausage and beef. Cook the meat, stirring to break it apart, until browned and cooked through, about 15 minutes. Season with 2 teaspoons of the salt. Drain all but 1 tablespoon of the fat, then transfer the meat and remaining fat to a large bowl and set aside to cool.

3. Put the eggs, cream cheese, sour cream, and the remaining ½ teaspoon of salt in a blender and blend until smooth.

4. Pour the egg mixture into the bowl of meat and stir to combine. Pour the mixture into the prepared casserole dish.

5. Bake until cooked through but still slightly jiggly in the center, about 45 minutes. Be careful not to overcook the casserole. It can be sliced and served right away or set aside to cool slightly, if you prefer.

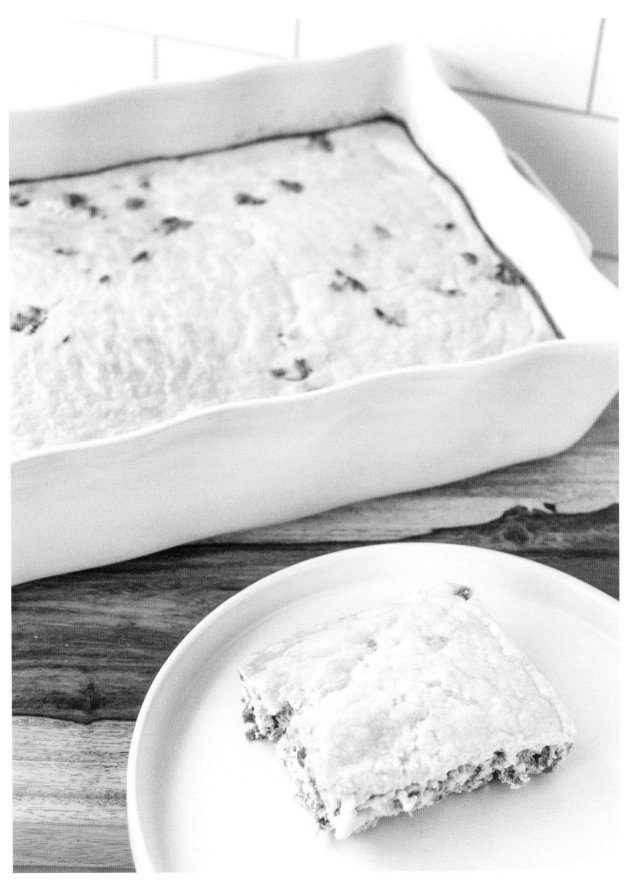

instant pot bacon and gruyère egg bites

YIELD:
7 bites (2 servings)

PREP TIME:
10 minutes (not including time to cook bacon)

COOK TIME:
9 minutes

This is my take on the yummy little egg bites from Starbucks, minus the gums, starches, carrageenan, and other not-ideal ingredients. These will make your life easier on busy mornings. Grab, heat, and go or even eat them cold—both ways are delicious. Aside from the Instant Pot, this recipe requires an egg bite mold and a trivet fitted to your Instant Pot. Speaking from experience, the most important tip I have to share is to be sure to use the lid that comes with the egg bite mold when cooking the egg bites. It may pop off a bit, but it will still be doing its job of keeping the portions bite-sized. Not using the lid will result in hugely expanded eggs on steroids, which is a wild ride you don't want to take.

4 large eggs

4 ounces (½ cup) cream cheese

¼ cup heavy cream

½ cup shredded Gruyère cheese (about 2 ounces)

½ teaspoon kosher salt

3 slices regular, thin-cut bacon, cooked (see page 166) and chopped

special equipment:
1 (7-well) silicone egg bite mold, plus trivet fitted for Instant Pot

1. Put all the ingredients, minus the bacon, in a blender and blend until smooth.

2. Distribute the chopped bacon among the wells of the egg bite mold.

3. Pour the batter over the bacon, filling each well to the top.

4. Secure the lid onto the mold, set the mold on the trivet, and lower it into the Instant Pot.

5. Add 1 cup of water, secure the Instant Pot lid, and select pressure cook on high heat for 9 minutes. Allow the pressure to release naturally for 10 minutes. After the natural release is completed, carefully flip the valve and release the rest of the pressure. Allow the egg bites to cool a bit before handling and enjoying.

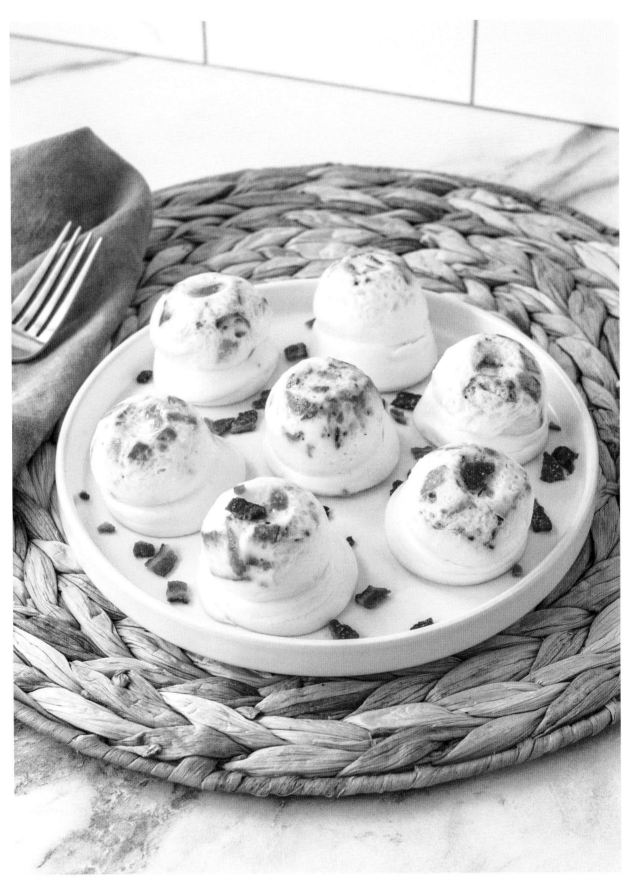

breakfast *of* champions

YIELD:
1 serving

PREP TIME:
5 minutes (not including time to cook steak and bacon)

COOK TIME:
4 minutes

The perfect breakfast to fill you up with all the nutrients you need to get your day started! The steak is quick to cook, and the bacon can be batch-cooked ahead of time to have on hand for breakfast. And forgive me for calling only for 2 to 3 slices of bacon. You have my permission to eat bacon to your heart's content.

1 tablespoon salted butter, for the pan

2 large eggs

Kosher salt

6 ounces Pan-Seared Skirt Steak (page 152)

2 to 3 slices regular, thin-cut bacon, cooked (see page 166)

1. Preheat a small skillet over medium heat until hot but not yet smoking.

2. When the pan is hot, drop in the butter and swirl to coat.

3. Crack the eggs into the pan and cook for 2 to 3 minutes on one side, flip and cook for 1 more minute for cooked-through whites and a runny yolk. Season with a light sprinkle of salt.

4. Serve immediately with the steak and bacon.

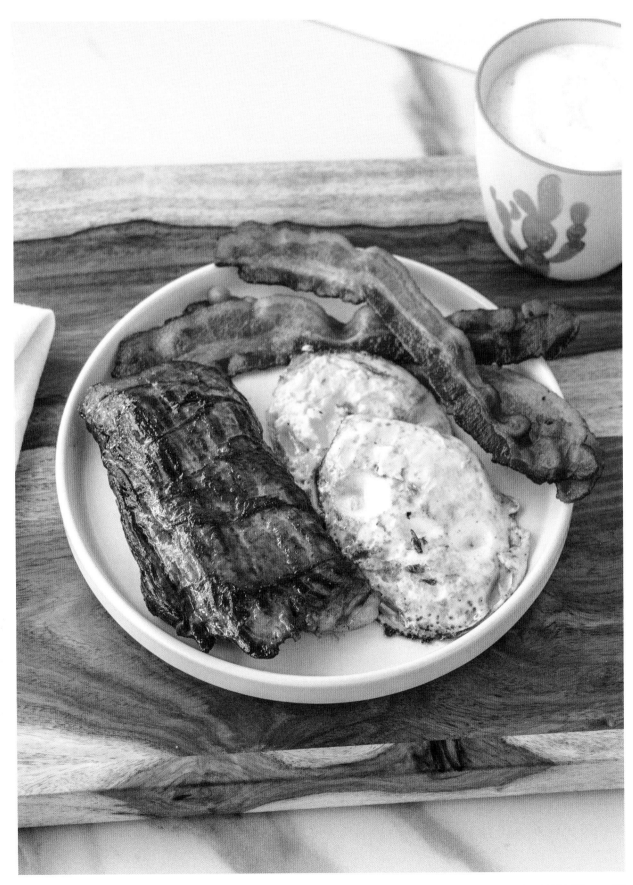

eggs benedict

YIELD:
4 servings

PREP TIME:
10 minutes (not including time to make muffins and sauce or cook bacon)

COOK TIME:
12 minutes

Eggs Benny isn't just for ordering at restaurants. It's easier to make at home than you think! Planning ahead and doing some prep work will make this gourmet meal a breeze to create. I suggest making the English muffins ahead of time—even the day before is fine. You can also cook the bacon a day in advance, but if you do it the day of, make it your first task and use my foolproof oven method (see page 166). While the bacon is baking, make the hollandaise sauce. When it's ready, you'll need to keep it warm and use it within an hour or two. After sitting, it may need a little blending before serving. The last step is to poach the eggs!

Distilled white vinegar, for the poaching water

8 large eggs

4 English muffins (page 84), cut in half and toasted

8 slices regular, thin-cut bacon, cooked (see page 166) and cut in half crosswise, plus extra crumbled cooked bacon for garnish, if desired

1 batch Hollandaise Sauce (page 208), for serving

1. To poach the eggs, fill a medium-size pot or pan with water and bring to a simmer. The ideal vessel will be wider than it is tall—deep enough to hold about 3 inches of water and wide enough to poach two eggs at a time, such as a shallow soup pot or deep sauté pan. A large saucepan filled halfway with water will also work. Add a splash of vinegar to the poaching water to help the whites hold their shape.

2. Crack an egg into a ramekin. Stir the water with the handle of a long wooden spoon to create a little whirlpool. Gently slide the egg from the ramekin into the center of the whirlpool. Repeat with another egg, poaching 2 eggs at a time. Simmer for 2 to 3 minutes, until the whites are set and the yolks are still runny. Remove the poached eggs to a dish of warm water.

3. Repeat with the remaining eggs.

4. Before serving, scoop the eggs onto a paper towel–lined plate, draining the excess liquid and picking off any funky white pieces.

5. To assemble: Arrange the two halves of a toasted English muffin on a serving plate. Top each half with two bacon pieces, followed by an egg, and finally some hollandaise sauce. Garnish with crumbled bacon, if desired. Repeat with the remaining ingredients.

6. Serve immediately and enjoy.

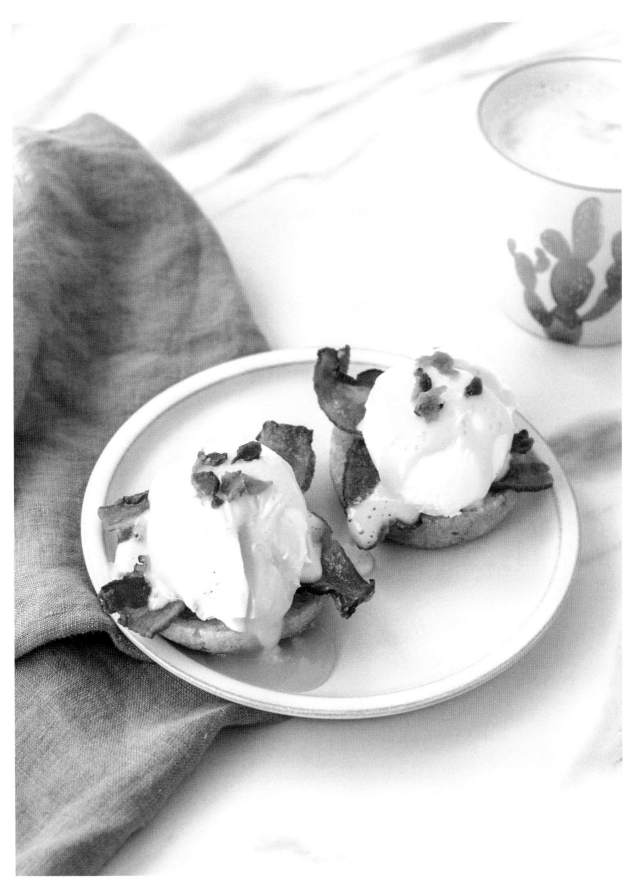

breakfast burrito

YIELD:
1 burrito

PREP TIME:
5 minutes (not including time to cook bacon and tortilla)

COOK TIME:
5 minutes

While I do love the classic bacon-and-eggs breakfast, there's just something so satisfying about sinking your teeth into a nice, hearty burrito. You won't even realize the tortillas don't have carbs. These would also be great to meal prep for the week. Just heat, grab, and go!

2 large eggs

1 tablespoon heavy cream

1 tablespoon salted butter, for the pan

Kosher salt

1 slice cheese (any type)

2 slices regular, thin-cut bacon, cooked (see page 166)

1 (7- to 8-inch) Tortilla (page 88)

1. Preheat a small skillet over medium-low heat.

2. While the pan is heating, crack the eggs into a small bowl and add the cream. Whisk well.

3. When the pan is hot, drop in the butter and swirl to coat the pan. Pour in the eggs and stir constantly, slowly cooking them over gentle heat so they stay super creamy. Sprinkle lightly with salt.

4. Once the eggs are set, about 2 minutes, turn off the heat.

5. Place the cheese slice on the eggs and cover the pan for 2 minutes.

6. To assemble the burrito, place the bacon in the center of the tortilla, then top the bacon with the cheesy eggs. Roll the tortilla into an open-ended burrito by folding one side in halfway, then folding up the bottom, and then folding the other side over. Serve immediately.

Note:

If making several burritos at once for meal prep, wrap each burrito with parchment paper and then foil or plastic wrap to hold it closed. Store in the refrigerator for up to 5 days. To rewarm a burrito, remove the foil or plastic, keep the parchment paper on, and microwave until heated through, about 1 minute.

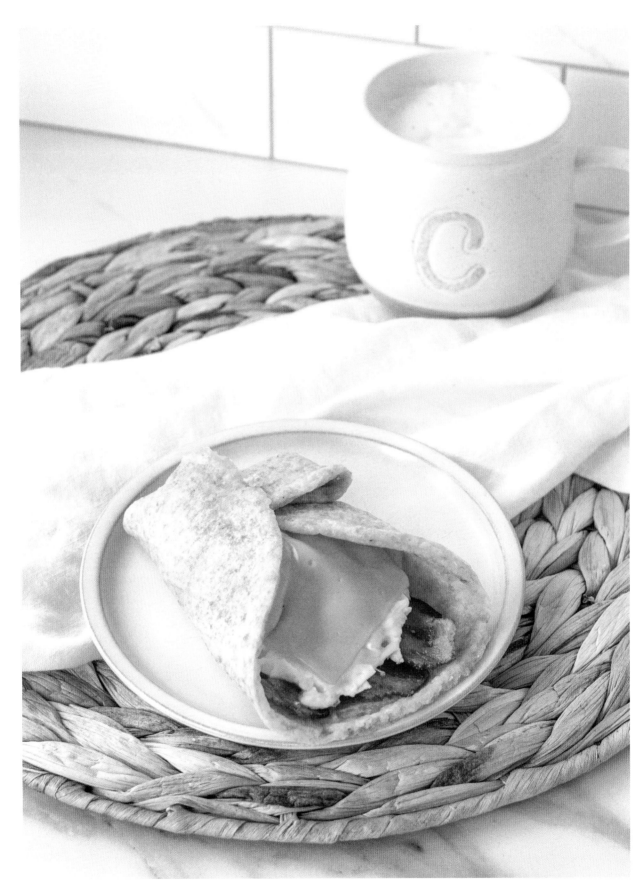

prosciutto egg cups

YIELD:
6 egg cups (2 to 3 servings)

PREP TIME:
10 minutes

COOK TIME:
25 minutes

I love a well-rounded little meal that is perfect for meal prep and reheats deliciously. These egg cups are great for those who are not using spices because, unlike salami, prosciutto typically does not contain spices. Plus, there's something about prosciutto that makes me feel rich and fancy when I eat it. Make your mornings easier or impress your brunch guests with these little cuties. To make them even more special, garnish them with a touch of smoked salt.

6 slices prosciutto (about 3 ounces)

¾ cup shredded cheese, such as cheddar (about 3 ounces)

6 large eggs

Smoked salt or kosher salt, for garnish

Chopped cooked bacon, for garnish (optional)

special equipment:
Standard-size 12-well silicone muffin pan

1. Preheat the oven to 375°F.

2. Take a slice of prosciutto and line one well of the muffin pan, covering the bottom and sides thoroughly to keep the egg and cheese from seeping through the prosciutto and sticking to the pan. Repeat with the remaining slices of prosciutto to make 6 cups.

3. Place 2 tablespoons of cheese in each prosciutto cup, then crack an egg into each cup.

4. Bake for 25 minutes, or until the eggs are medium-cooked (the yolks will be just set and creamy).

5. Top with a sprinkle of salt—smoked salt if you're feeling wild—and, if desired, some chopped bacon.

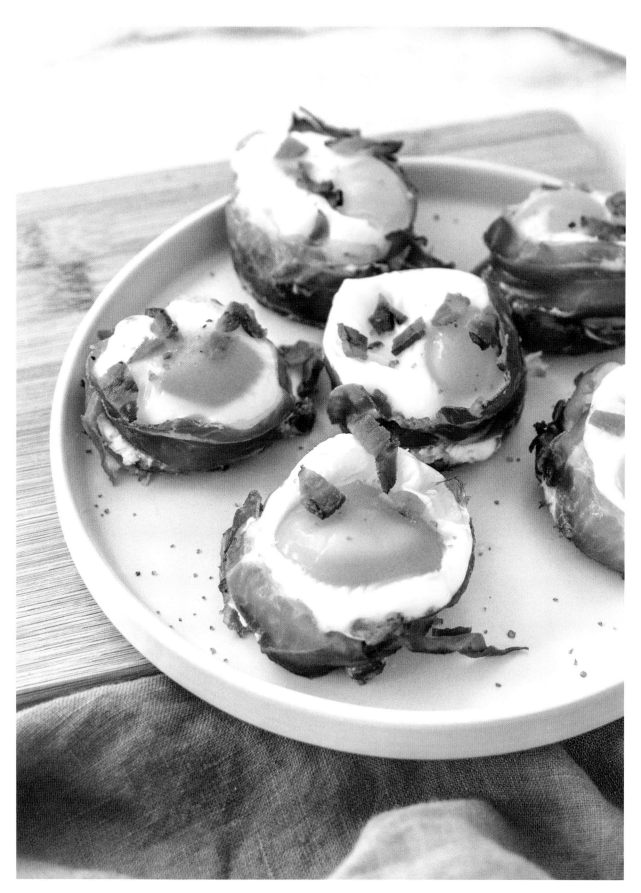

breakfast meatballs

YIELD:
12 (2½-inch) meatballs
(3 to 4 servings)

PREP TIME:
10 minutes

COOK TIME:
20 minutes

Who doesn't love an easy breakfast? These meatballs are great to prep ahead of time and pop in the oven in the morning. You can also cook them in an air fryer (see the note below). Serve them up with a creamy coffee, and you're in for a delight.

1 pound bulk breakfast sausage (see notes)

3 ounces (6 tablespoons) cream cheese, softened

1 large egg

1 cup shredded Parmesan cheese (about 4 ounces)

1. Preheat the oven to 400°F.

2. Put all the ingredients in a large bowl and mix well with your hands.

3. Separate the mixture into 12 equal portions and roll them into balls. The mixture will be wet and will not form perfectly.

4. Place the meatballs on a sheet pan and bake for 16 to 20 minutes, until cooked through and golden brown on top. When done, they will no longer be pink in the center and the internal temperature will be 160°F.

 Notes:

Please be aware of the ingredients in breakfast sausage and read the labels carefully. Breakfast sausage contains seasonings, so if you are not using any, use ground pork instead. Another thing to pay attention to is added ingredients like sugar and oils that you may want to avoid. Look for brands that list only pork and seasonings on the label.

To make these meatballs in an air fryer, preheat the air fryer to 400°F on the oven setting and bake for 18 to 20 minutes, until browned and cooked through. When done, they will no longer be pink in the center, and the internal temperature will be 160°F.

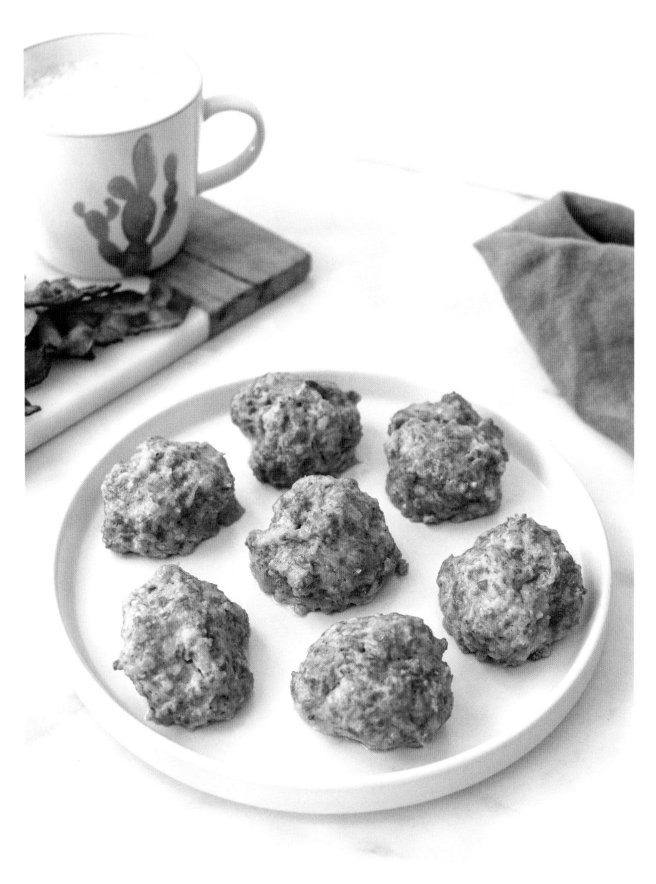

cottage cheese eggs

YIELD:
2 servings

PREP TIME:
5 minutes

COOK TIME:
5 minutes

Add some extra protein and creaminess to your morning eggs with cottage cheese! We often use cream cheese or shredded cheese for our scrambles, but there's something unique and delicious about using cottage cheese, and you can't beat the high protein. This scramble is also great to serve up for guests; just double or triple the recipe as needed.

4 large eggs

½ cup cottage cheese

1 tablespoon salted butter, for the pan

Kosher salt

1. Preheat a medium-size skillet over medium heat.

2. Crack the eggs into a medium-size bowl and whisk until the whites and yolks are combined.

3. Add the cottage cheese to the bowl and whisk until the eggs and cottage cheese are well blended.

4. Drop the butter into the pan, swirl to coat, then add the egg and cheese mixture.

5. Cook, stirring occasionally to scramble, until the eggs are set and the cottage cheese is melted, about 5 minutes.

6. Add salt to taste and serve immediately.

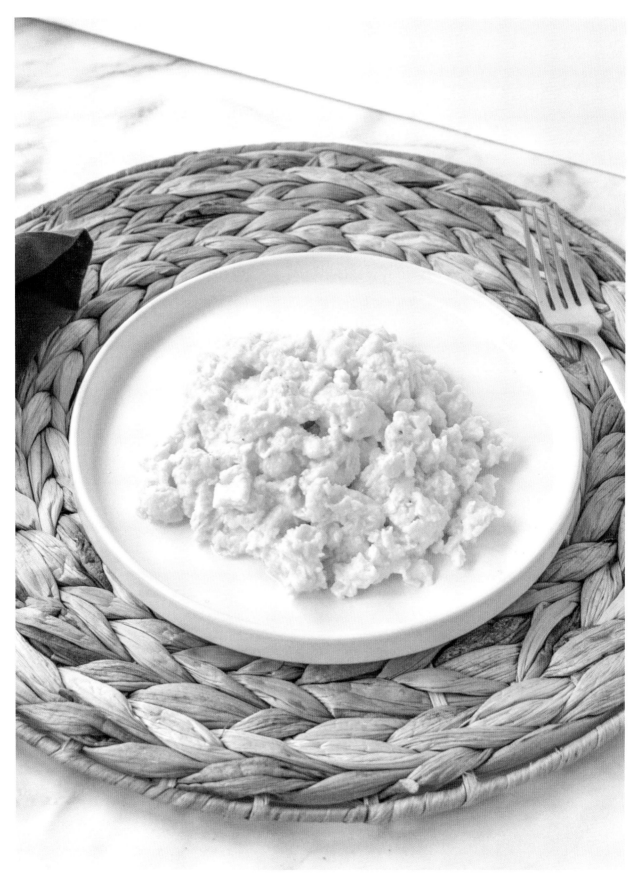

biscuits *and* gravy

YIELD:
4 to 6 servings

PREP TIME:
5 minutes (not including time to make muffins)

COOK TIME:
15 minutes

When I was cooking on yachts, this was one of my favorite meals to make when we were underway doing a boat delivery. When you're at sea for days on end, having a hot and comforting breakfast works magic on cranky sailors. Granted, we weren't using pork rind biscuits, and the gravy had a flour-based roux, but I think the crew would love this new version.

FOR THE GRAVY:
(Makes 3 cups)

1 tablespoon tallow or other heat-tolerant fat of choice, for the pan

1 pound bulk breakfast sausage (see note, page 68)

1 cup heavy cream

4 ounces (½ cup) cream cheese

4 to 6 English Muffins (page 84), sliced in half, for serving

1. Preheat a large skillet over medium-high heat until hot and just beginning to smoke.

2. Drop in the tallow and swirl to coat the pan. Add the sausage and brown, stirring occasionally to break it apart, until cooked through, 8 to 10 minutes. Drain all but 1 tablespoon of the fat.

3. Pour in the cream and add the cream cheese. Stir until the cheese is incorporated, then continue to cook for 3 to 4 minutes, stirring occasionally, to warm and thicken the gravy.

4. Serve immediately over the English muffins.

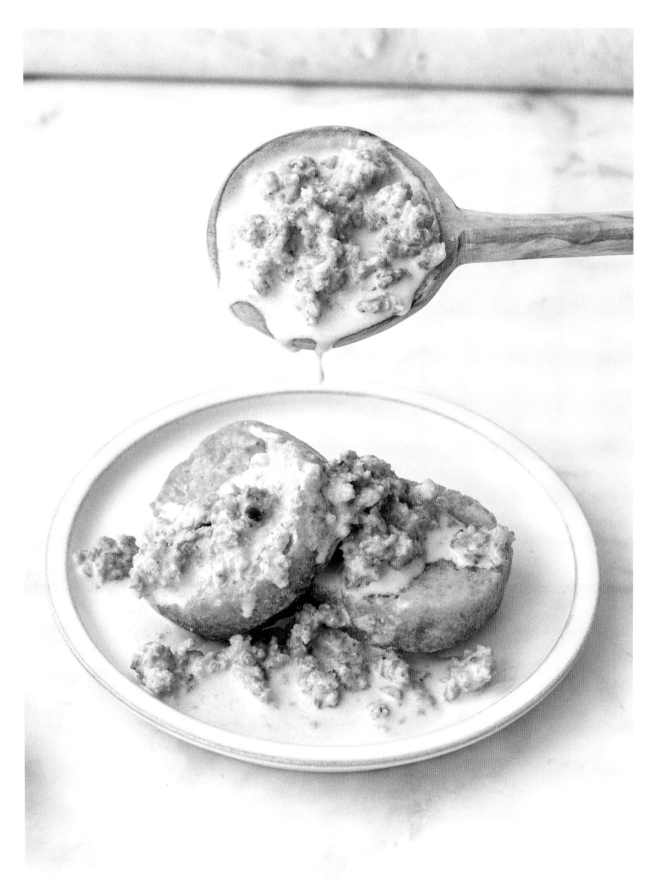

mini bagels

YIELD:
3 mini bagels (2 to 3 servings)

PREP TIME:
10 minutes

COOK TIME:
18 minutes

OK, look. We all know these aren't going to be like a freshly baked NYC bagel, but you can't blame a gal for trying. I think they're close, and when you haven't had a bagel in years, well, you could spread cream cheese on a piece of cardboard, and it would be satisfying. That being said, my kids (who have been to the dark side and have eaten gluten-filled bagels) really like these and eat them with joy in their eyes. They're like little Gordon Ramsays, so if they approve of these bagels, then they deserve a five-star rating in my book.

1½ cups shredded mozzarella cheese (about 6 ounces)

1 ounce (2 tablespoons) cream cheese, softened

1 large egg, whisked

¾ cup (68 grams) pork panko

Cream cheese, for serving

special equipment:
1 (6-cavity) silicone donut/mini bagel pan

1. Preheat the oven to 400°F.

2. Put the mozzarella, cream cheese, egg, and panko in a medium-size microwave-safe bowl and mix well.

3. Microwave for 90 seconds on high power, stopping to stir in 30-second increments, until the cheese is fully melted.

4. Continue to stir the mixture until you have a cohesive dough; as you work the dough, it will cool and start to firm up. At that point, you may want to switch to your hands to knead the dough, or you can continue working it (vigorously) with the spoon.

5. Once you have a cohesive ball of dough, separate it into 3 equal portions and then roll each piece between your hands to form an 8-inch-long rope.

6. Put a dough rope in a cavity in the donut pan and pinch the ends together to join them. Repeat with the other two dough ropes.

7. Bake until the bagels are well browned, 15 to 18 minutes.

8. To serve, slice in half and toast or broil to get crispy. Top with cream cheese.

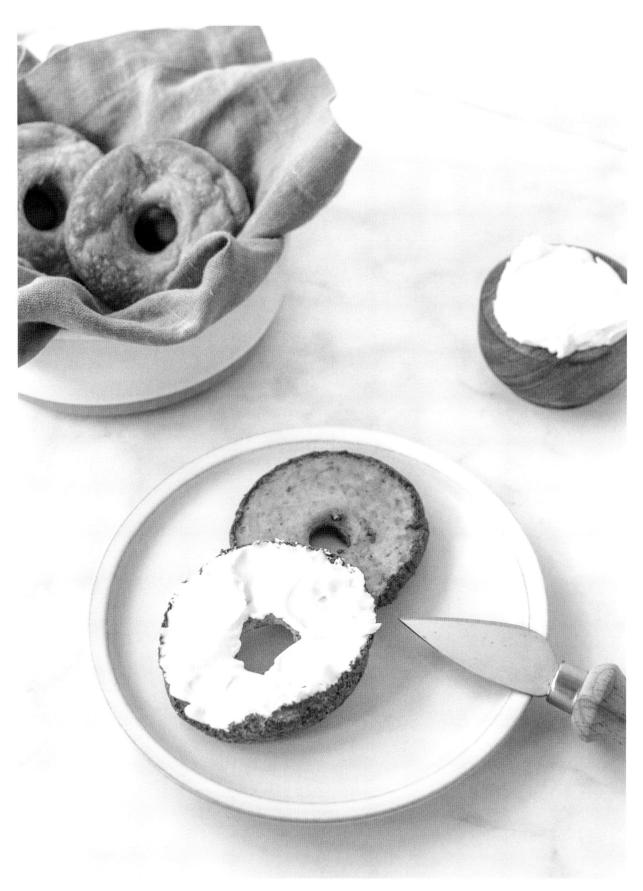

dutch baby soufflé

YIELD:
8 servings

PREP TIME:
10 minutes

COOK TIME:
30 minutes

This recipe was an accidental blessing. I was trying to make a loaf of bread, but it wasn't dry enough. However, it was still delicious, so I added some cinnamon and vanilla and ran with it! Think French toast meets bread pudding, then fist bumps a soufflé and high-fives a Dutch baby (the German pancake, not an infant). If you're confused about what you just read, it's OK; so am I. And if you're feeling extra wild, see the note below on how to kick it up an extra notch.

½ cup (1 stick) salted butter, melted

½ cup heavy cream

½ cup unflavored, unsweetened protein powder

½ cup egg white powder

4 large eggs

1 (8-ounce) package cream cheese

1 tablespoon unflavored powdered gelatin

¼ teaspoon kosher salt

1 teaspoon vanilla extract

1¼ teaspoons ground cinnamon, divided

1. Preheat the oven to 375°F. Line the bottom and sides of an 8-inch square baking pan with parchment paper.

2. Place all the ingredients except ¼ teaspoon of the cinnamon in a food processor and blend well. Pour into the prepared pan.

3. Sprinkle the remaining ¼ teaspoon of cinnamon onto the top and swirl it with a toothpick.

4. Bake until cooked through and lightly browned, about 30 minutes. To test doneness, insert a toothpick in the center—it should come out clean. The Dutch baby will puff up a lot but will deflate once removed from the oven.

5. Cut into 8 slices and serve immediately, or slice and air-fry until crispy, following the instruction in the note below. Leftovers should be rewarmed before eating.

Note:

I love eating this fresh from the oven, but there's something extra delicious about getting it crispy. The air fryer is perfect for this task. Take a slice and cut it horizontally to expose the center. Then pop it into the air fryer preheated to 400°F and toast for 3 to 5 minutes on each side, until crispy. Spread a light layer of salted butter on top before enjoying. If you don't have an air fryer, a toaster oven works well, too.

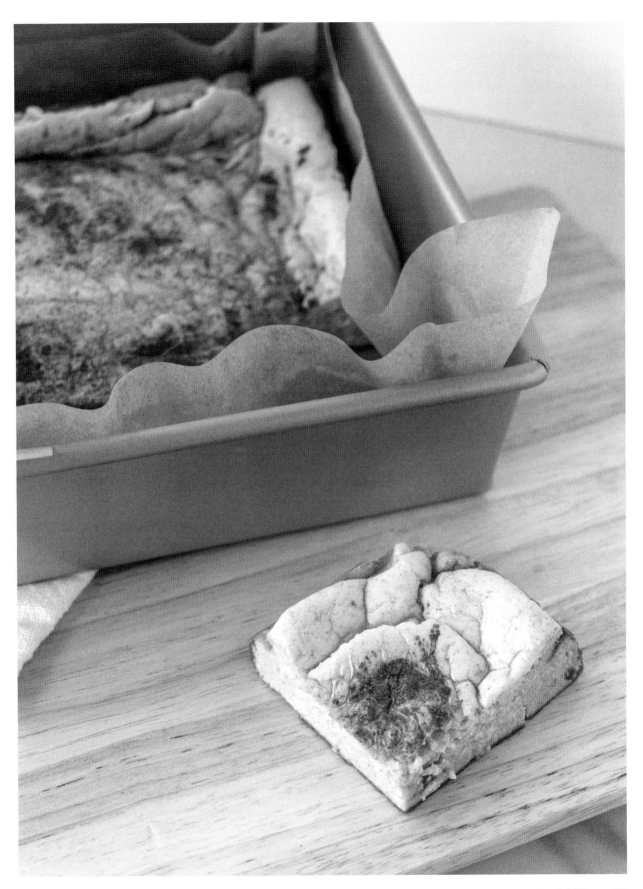

cinnamon rolls

YIELD:
8 rolls (8 servings)

PREP TIME:
15 minutes

COOK TIME:
40 minutes

My family always enjoys cinnamon rolls on Christmas morning, and with this version, we can have them and still be healthy. My kids love them, which says a lot because they've had regular gluten- and sugar-filled cinnamon rolls in the past. Mom win! I often say you can skip the cinnamon and vanilla if you're a strict carnivore, but don't do that with these. You'd probably be disappointed with the flavor. If you're eating carnivore due to autoimmune issues, you may want to skip these (in the beginning, at least) because of the spices and enjoy one of my Mini Bagels (page 74) instead—the dough is the same except for the vanilla.

FOR THE DOUGH:

3 cups shredded mozzarella cheese (about 12 ounces)

2 ounces (¼ cup) cream cheese, softened

2 large eggs, whisked

1½ cups (135 grams) pork panko

1 teaspoon vanilla extract

FOR THE FILLING:

¼ cup (½ stick) salted butter, softened

1 tablespoon ground cinnamon, plus extra for garnish

FOR THE FROSTING:

4 ounces (½ cup) cream cheese, softened

¼ cup (½ stick) salted butter, softened

½ teaspoon vanilla extract

1. Preheat the oven to 350°F.

2. To make the dough, place all the ingredients in a large microwave-safe bowl and mix well.

3. Microwave for 3 to 4 minutes on high power, stirring at 30-second intervals, until all the cheese is melted.

4. Continue to stir the mixture until you have a cohesive dough; as you work the dough, it will cool and start to firm up. At that point, you may want to switch to your hands to knead the dough, or you can continue working it (vigorously) with the spoon.

5. Take the dough and place it on a large piece of parchment paper (at least 16 inches long). Using your hands, press and shape the dough until it is about 12 by 15 inches. Let cool.

6. Spread the softened butter on the dough, making sure to cover the entire surface, including the edges. Sprinkle the cinnamon evenly over the butter.

7. Working from the long side, roll the dough into a log and cut into 8 pieces.

8. Place the rolls cut side up in a 9-inch cake pan and bake until golden brown, 35 to 40 minutes.

9. Mix the frosting ingredients together in a small bowl. Spread onto the rolls, garnish with a little sprinkle of cinnamon, and serve warm. Gently rewarm leftover rolls before eating, being careful not to overheat them or the frosting will melt.

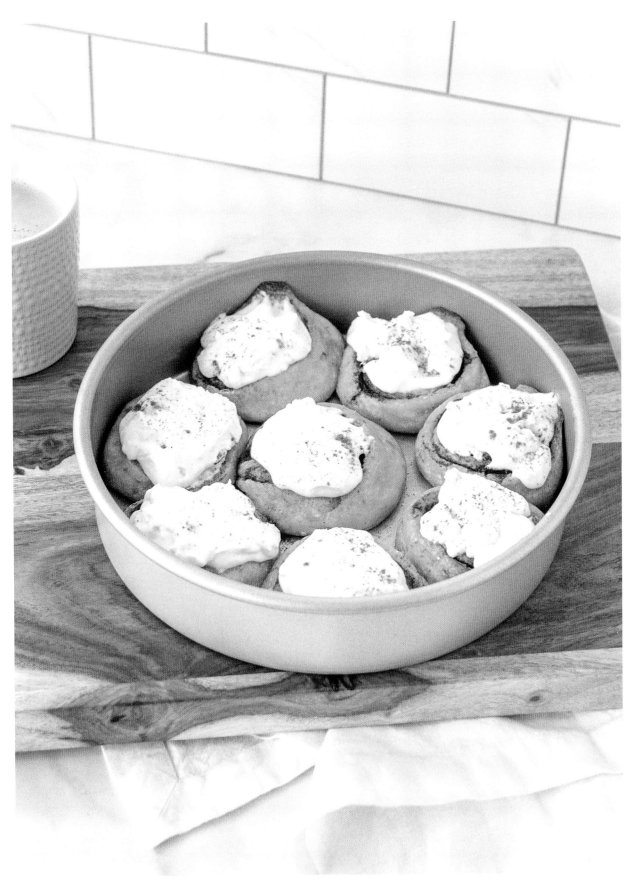

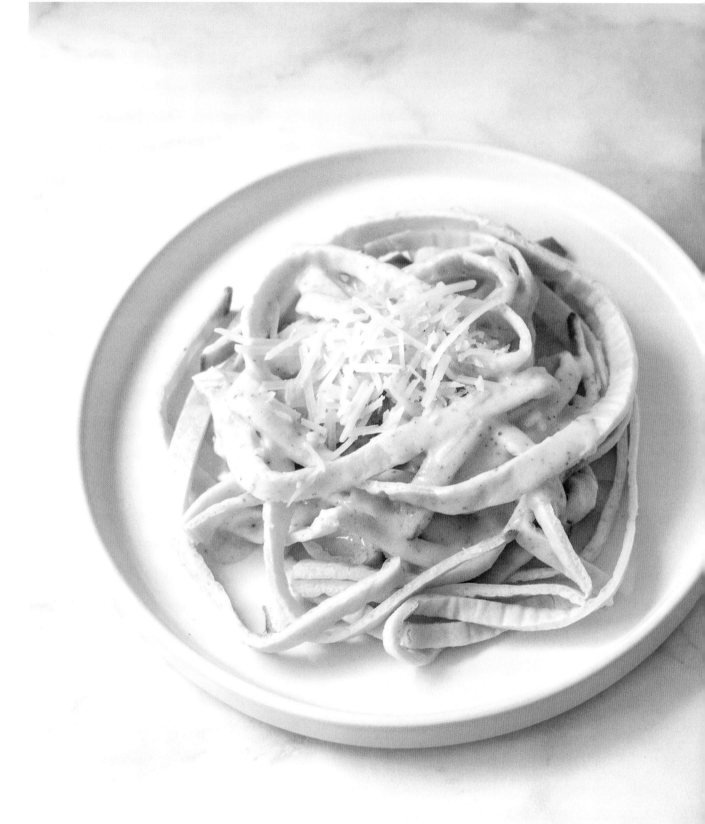

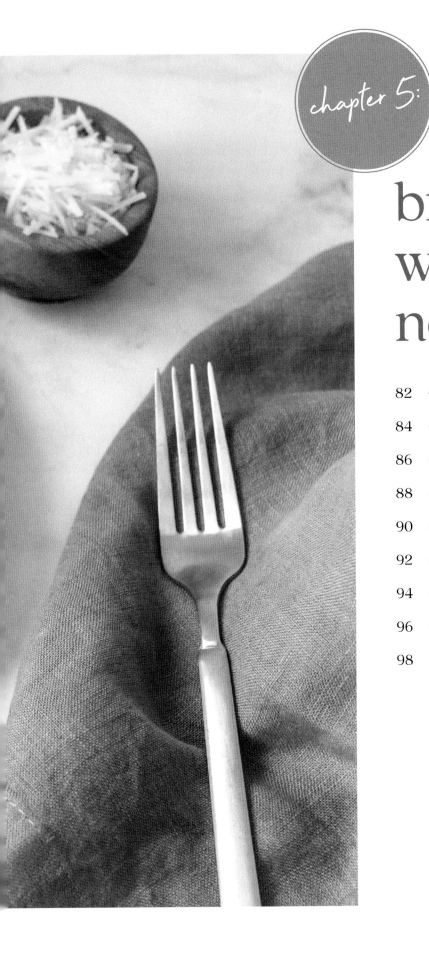

breads, wraps & noodles

carnivore bread

YIELD:
1 loaf (22 slices slightly less than ½ inch thick, 11 servings)

PREP TIME:
10 minutes

COOK TIME:
1 hour

This bread is perfect for morning toast with butter or your favorite sandwich goodies. The texture is like banana bread, and while that's delicious as is, I love toasting it in an air fryer preheated to 425°F for about 10 minutes (flipping halfway). If you don't have an air fryer, a toaster oven works, too. Toasting dries it out a bit and gives it a more traditional toasted bread texture. It's also lovely pan-fried in butter on a skillet and topped with a sprinkle of cinnamon, which gives it the texture and flavor of French toast. If you have leftover bread that you won't get to within four or five days, pop it in the freezer; it freezes beautifully!

12 large eggs

1½ cups cottage cheese

2 cups (180 grams) pork panko

½ cup (1 stick) salted butter, melted

1. Preheat the oven to 375°F. Line a 9 by 5-inch loaf pan with parchment paper, allowing the paper to extend over the edges of the pan for easy removal.

2. Put the eggs, cottage cheese, panko, and butter in a food processor and blend until smooth.

3. Pour the batter into the prepared pan and bake until browned and a toothpick comes out clean when inserted in the middle, about 1 hour.

4. Let cool for a bit before removing from the pan. Allow the bread to cool completely before slicing. For the best texture, toast slices before serving (see note, above).

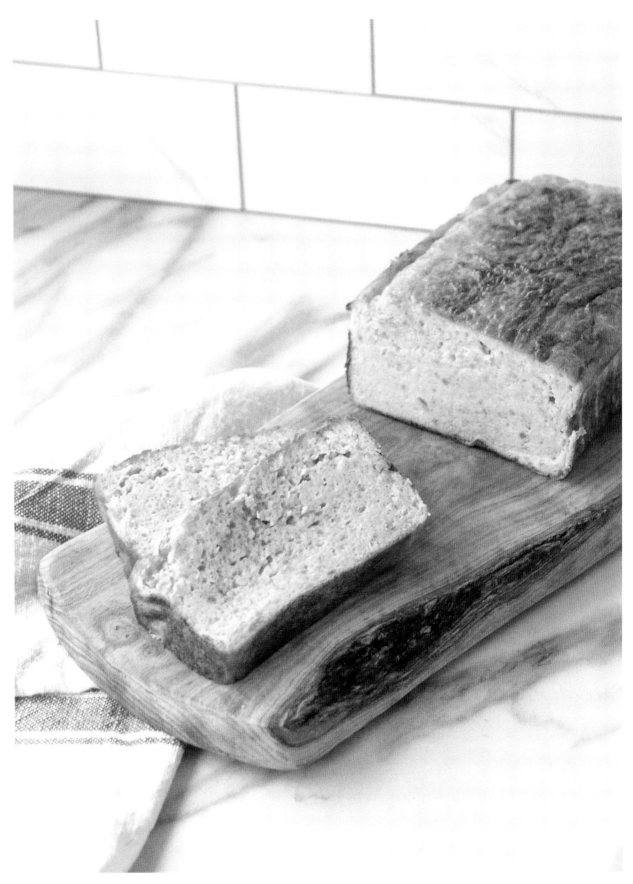

english muffins

YIELD:
12 muffins (6 to 12 servings)

PREP TIME:
10 minutes

COOK TIME:
20 minutes

Sometimes you just need to sink your teeth into something with the texture of bread! These savory muffins are delicious straight out of the oven, sliced and toasted and used for Eggs Benedict (page 62), or as a stand-in for biscuits in my Biscuits and Gravy recipe (page 72). You can even use them as little buns for sliders.

2 cups (180 grams) pork panko

8 large eggs

¼ cup (½ stick) salted butter, melted but not hot

special equipment:
Standard-size 12-well silicone muffin pan

1. Preheat the oven to 400°F.

2. Put the panko, eggs, and butter in a large bowl and mix well with a fork until the ingredients are incorporated into a moderately thick batter.

3. Spoon the batter into the muffin pan, filling the wells about three-quarters full.

4. Bake for 18 to 20 minutes, until the muffins are browned and a toothpick comes out clean when inserted in the middle.

5. Let the muffins cool slightly in the pan, until you can comfortably handle them, then pop them out and serve warm. Rewarm leftovers before eating.

Note:
I recommend using a silicone muffin pan so the muffins can be removed easily without sticking.

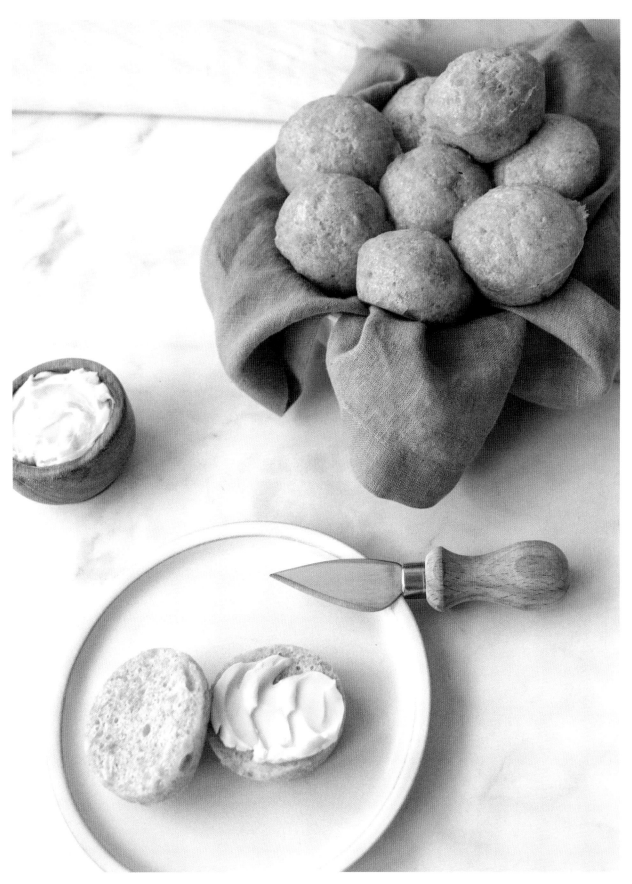

all-purpose waffles

YIELD:
6 to 8 mini waffles
(3 to 4 servings)

PREP TIME:
5 minutes

COOK TIME:
18 to 24 minutes, depending
on yield

Early in my carnivore days, I watched a video on the YouTube channel Living Life Now that explains how to make pork rind bread. I tweaked that recipe to come up with these waffles, and over the years I've experimented with this basic batter to make my own versions of biscuits, tortillas, and more.

These waffles are my go-to anytime I need bread for a meal. Use them as burger buns and sandwich bread or make them your next favorite breakfast treat, jazzed up with vanilla, cinnamon, and whipped cream (see the variation below). The yield varies between six and eight waffles depending on the exact size of your mini waffle maker and the amount of batter it holds. Mine makes eight 4-inch waffles.

1 cup (90 grams) pork panko

4 large eggs, whisked

¼ cup (½ stick) salted butter, melted but not hot

special equipment:
Nonstick mini waffle maker

1. Preheat a mini waffle maker according to the manufacturer's directions.

2. To make the batter, put the panko, eggs, and butter in a medium-size bowl and mix well with a fork until the ingredients are incorporated into a moderately thick batter.

3. Take a small scoop of the batter and drop it onto the waffle iron. (See the waffle manufacturer's instructions for recommended quantity; my waffle maker holds about 3 tablespoons.) Spread the batter to the edges, making sure that all the grooves and peaks are covered.

4. Cook the waffle for 2 to 3 minutes, until toasty and browned. Repeat with the remaining batter to make a total of 6 to 8 waffles.

Variation:

Breakfast Waffles. *Add 1 teaspoon vanilla extract and ½ teaspoon ground cinnamon to the batter in Step 2. Garnish the waffles with whipped cream, if desired.*

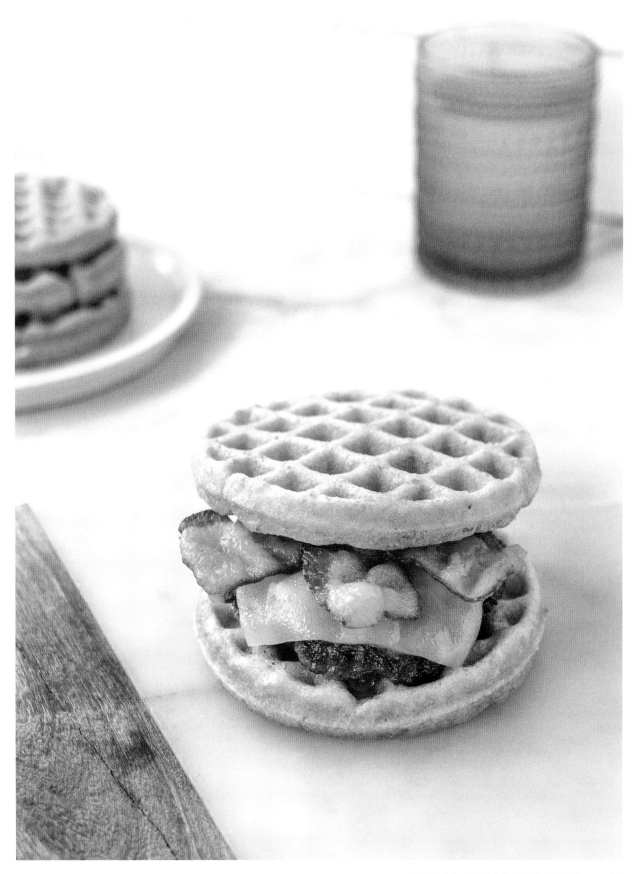

tortillas

YIELD:
Eight 6-inch or six 7- to 8-inch tortillas (4 servings)

PREP TIME:
10 minutes

COOK TIME:
24 minutes

Have a fiesta with these carnivore tortillas! You won't even notice that they don't have flour in them. OK, that may be pushing it, but when the whole family loves them (mine does!), it's a huge win. These are great to make ahead of time for meal prep. The smaller 6-inch tortillas are perfect for soft tacos and quesadillas, and the larger 7- to 8-inch ones are best for burritos, such as my Breakfast Burrito on page 64. For this recipe, you need either a burger smasher/press (for 6-inch tortillas) or a waffle cone iron (for 7- to 8-inch ones) to press the batter to the perfect thickness. Note that waffle cone irons range in size from 7 to 8 inches; mine is 7½ inches.

1 cup (90 grams) pork panko

4 large eggs, whisked

¼ cup (½ stick) salted butter, melted but not hot

Tallow or other heat-tolerant fat of choice, for the pan and burger smasher/press

special equipment:
Burger smasher/press at least 5½ inches in diameter, or nonstick waffle cone iron

1. If making 6-inch tortillas, preheat a medium-size skillet over medium-high heat and have a burger smasher/press on hand. If making 7- to 8-inch tortillas, preheat a waffle cone iron.

2. Put the panko, eggs, and butter in a medium-size bowl and mix well with a fork until the ingredients are incorporated into a moderately thick batter. If making the larger size tortillas, skip ahead to Step 6.

3. To make the smaller tortillas, grease the burger smasher with tallow, then grease the hot pan with tallow. Place a little less than ¼ cup of the batter in the center of the pan.

4. Immediately press down on the thick batter with the greased burger smasher to make a thin layer about 6 inches in diameter. Leave the burger smasher in place for 1 to 2 minutes before flipping the tortilla to cook the other side. When the tortilla peels off the burger smasher easily and is browned, it's ready to be flipped. Once flipped, cook for another minute, until golden brown on both sides.

5. Repeat with the rest of the batter, regreasing the burger smasher as needed, making a total of 8 tortillas.

6. To make the larger tortillas, place ¼ cup of the batter onto the waffle cone iron and press down until you have a thin layer of batter spread to the edges of the iron. Cook for about 2 minutes, or until golden brown. Repeat with the remaining batter.

7. Serve warm or at room temperature. If you have leftovers or have made extra for meal prep, allow refrigerated tortillas to come to room temperature on the counter before eating, or rewarm them in the microwave for about 10 seconds.

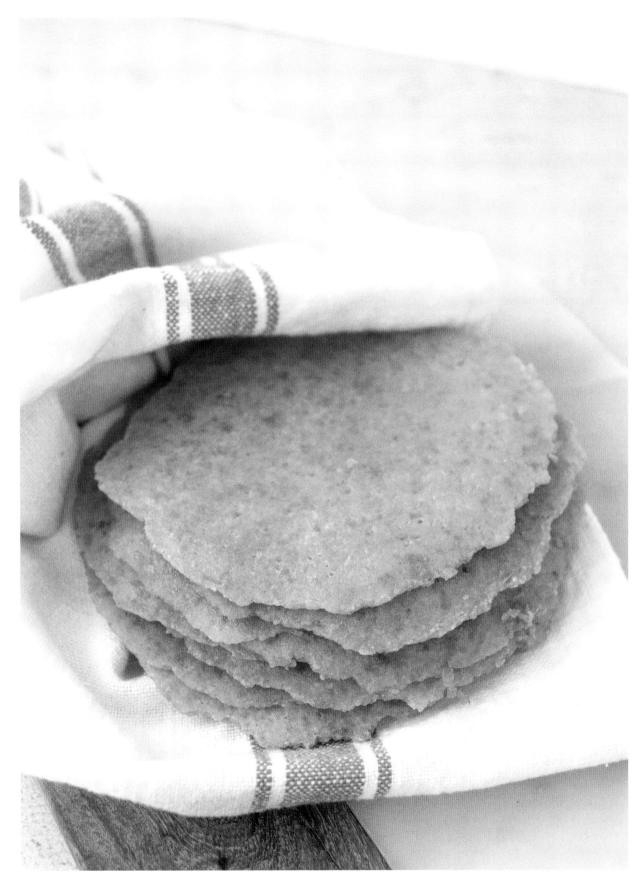

cornbread muffins

YIELD:
8 muffins (8 servings)

PREP TIME:
15 minutes

COOK TIME:
45 minutes

This version of an old-time comfort food makes me think I fell off the carnivore wagon! Let me tell you something about sweet corn extract, though: while it does give these muffins a corn flavor, it's not needed. And to be honest, it may not be great for some people. I wouldn't call it a perfectly clean ingredient, but it is low carb, and many people do fine with it. Most brands of corn extract include natural flavors, which can cause problems for some. In other words, use this ingredient at your discretion. I hope my note of caution hasn't scared you away from trying this recipe, because if you're looking for an accompaniment to my chili (see page 174), you can do no better than these muffins!

1 pound ground chicken

5 large eggs

1½ cups (135 grams) pork panko

¼ cup (½ stick) salted butter, softened (see note)

1 teaspoon sweet corn extract (optional)

1. Preheat the oven to 350°F. Line or grease 8 wells of a standard-size 12-well nonstick muffin pan.

2. Cook the ground chicken in a large skillet over medium-high heat, breaking it up as it cooks, until no longer pink; drain the cooking liquid. Allow the chicken to cool slightly before proceeding with the next step.

3. Put the chicken and remaining ingredients in a food processor and mix until combined; the batter will be slightly lumpy from the ground chicken.

4. Scoop the batter evenly into the prepared muffin wells, filling them to the top.

5. Bake for 30 minutes, or until browned and cooked through. To test doneness, insert a toothpick in the center of a muffin—it should come out clean.

6. Let cool for about 10 minutes before removing from the pan. These are best served warm. Rewarm leftovers before eating.

Note:

If you're following the Dairy-Free Carnivore Meal Plan (page 48), or you simply prefer these muffins to be dairy-free, replace the butter with ¼ cup softened tallow. If you store tallow at room temperature, the texture should be sufficiently soft as is.

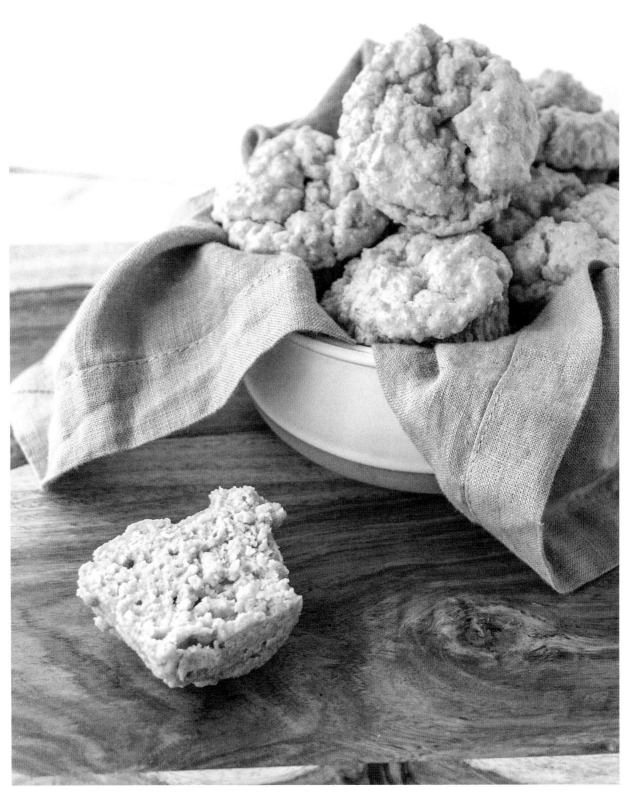

panko noodles

YIELD:
4 servings

PREP TIME:
10 minutes

COOK TIME:
20 minutes

Please don't tell the other recipes, but this is one of my favorites in this book. I mean, who doesn't love a nice big bowl of pasta? So comforting, delicious, and nutritious! Serve these noodles topped with your favorite sauce—I like my Browned Butter Cream Sauce (page 206)—and, if you wish, some shredded Parmesan cheese. For a heartier meal, top the noodles with sliced grilled chicken or steak.

4 large eggs

4 ounces (½ cup) cream cheese

¼ cup pork panko

2 tablespoons unflavored powdered gelatin

1. Preheat the oven to 350°F. Line a sheet pan with a silicone mat or parchment paper.

2. Put the eggs, cream cheese, panko, and gelatin in a blender and blend until smooth.

3. Pour the mixture onto the prepared pan and spread into a thin layer, almost to the edges. I find that using an offset spatula (for cake decorating) works best to get it flat and smooth.

4. Bake just until set and the edges have started to become lightly browned, about 20 minutes.

5. Slide the silicone mat or parchment paper with the sheet of noodle onto a cooling rack. Let cool until the sheet of noodle is still warm but you can comfortably handle it, about 10 minutes. This is a great time to get the sauce and Parmesan (if using) ready.

6. When cooled, loosely roll the sheet of noodle like you would a jelly roll, then slice crosswise into ribbons of your desired width.

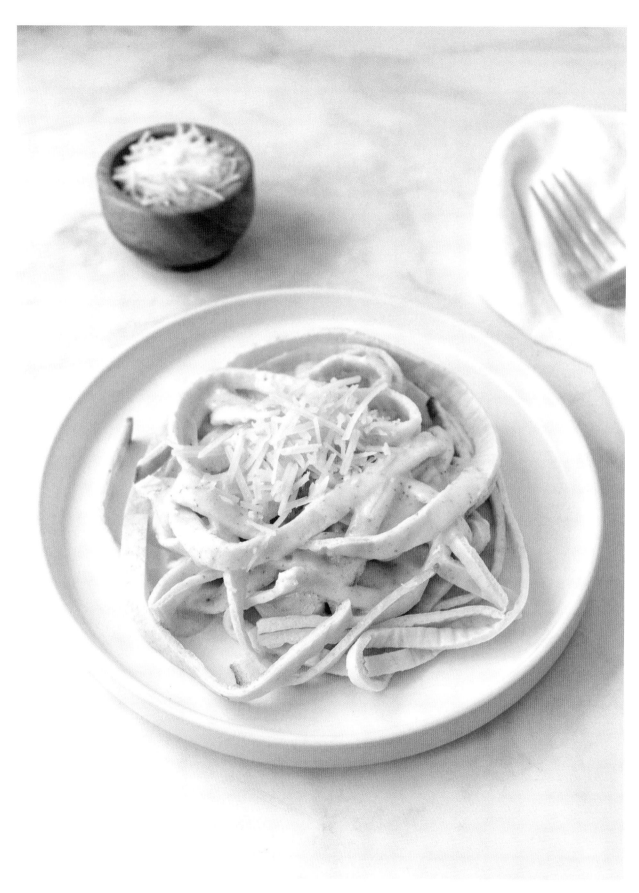

egg white noodles or wraps

YIELD:
1 to 2 servings noodles
or 3 wraps

PREP TIME:
5 minutes

COOK TIME:
5 minutes for noodles or
7½ minutes for wraps

This is a two-for-one recipe. You can use the same batter to make either noodles or wraps. If you're off pork or dairy, these noodles are a great alternative to my pork panko noodles on page 92. These pure protein noodles are great topped with your favorite sauce or protein, and you can't go wrong using them as wraps to wrap anything you like (my Chicken Salad on page 130 is a great choice). For a simple and light yet nourishing (though not dairy-free) meal, I like to top these noodles with Air Fryer Shrimp (page 142), a dollop of softened butter, and some shredded Parmesan.

½ cup egg whites (see notes)

1 tablespoon unflavored powdered gelatin

Pinch of kosher salt

1 tablespoon tallow, divided (for cooking the wraps)

1. *To make the batter,* combine the egg whites, gelatin, and salt in a small blender or mini food processor.

2. Blend until well combined, about 15 seconds. If you're making noodles, skip ahead to Step 7.

3. *To make wraps,* preheat a small skillet (7 to 8 inches in diameter) over medium heat. When hot, drop in a teaspoon of the tallow and swirl to coat the pan.

4. Pour one-third of the batter into the greased pan, and immediately swirl the pan so that the batter goes to the edges of the pan and you have a thin wrap.

5. Cook until the egg is set, about 2 minutes, then flip and cook for 30 seconds more.

6. Repeat with the remaining tallow and batter to make a total of 3 wraps. Can be used warm, at room temperature, or cold.

Notes:

For this quantity of egg whites, you'll need 4 or 5 large eggs. Save the leftover yolks for making other recipes in this book, such as Fried Egg Yolks (page 114), Hollandaise Sauce (page 208), Butter Bacon Mayonnaise (page 210), Carnivore Ice Cream—3 Ways (page 194), or Ice Cream Sandwiches (page 198). Raw egg yolks will keep for up to 2 days.

For the wraps, if you don't own a 7- to 8-inch skillet, you can use a medium-size skillet to make two wraps instead of three. If you'd like to end up with some wraps and noodles from the same batch of batter, you can roll up and slice one or two of the wraps into noodles. However, if you just want noodles, the hands-off oven method is a faster option.

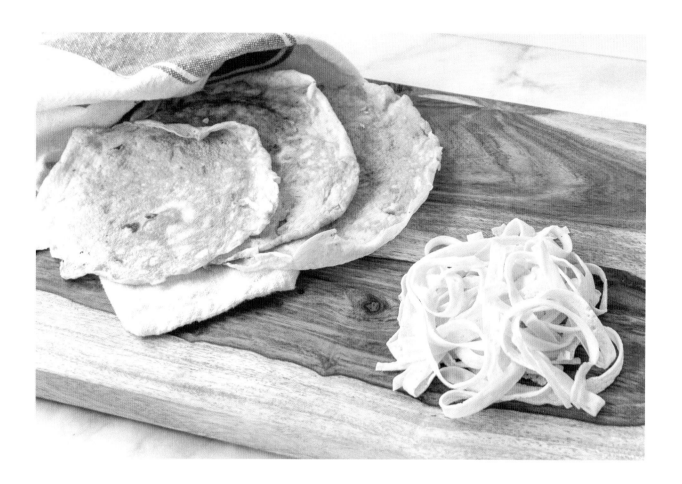

7. *To make noodles*, preheat the oven to 400°F and line a sheet pan with a silicone mat or parchment paper.

8. Pour the batter onto the prepared pan and use an offset spatula to spread it into a large thin rectangle, about ⅛ inch thick.

9. Bake for 5 minutes or until set.

10. Slide the liner with the noodle sheet onto a cooling rack. Let cool completely before removing the noodle sheet from the liner. If it is sticking, pop the liner into the freezer for a few minutes, and the sheet of noodle will peel off nicely. If you need to fold it over to make it fit in your freezer, that's fine.

11. To slice into noodles, roll the sheet like you would a jelly roll and then slice crosswise into ribbons of your desired width. You can keep the strips wide for use as lasagna noodles, or you can slice them into fettuccine-like noodles.

12. Before serving, rewarm the noodles in the microwave or in a dry or greased pan over moderate heat.

cheese wrap

YIELD:
1 wrap

PREP TIME:
1 minute

COOK TIME:
5 minutes

No need to miss your favorite sandwich anymore! Fill this cheese wrap with your favorites—Chicken Salad (page 130), bacon and eggs, your choice of deli meats with Butter Bacon Mayonnaise (page 210). These hold up great in the refrigerator, so they are a perfect item to meal prep for the week.

2 slices cheese, such as cheddar, each about 3 inches square

1. Line an appropriately sized sheet pan with parchment paper. If using an air fryer or toaster oven to make this wrap, grab a small sheet pan; if using a regular-size oven, any size sheet pan will do.

2. Place the cheese slices on the prepared pan, overlapping their edges slightly so they form one large rectangular piece.

3. Preheat the air fryer to 400°F on the oven setting. (Do not use the air fry setting; in some air fryers, the fan may blow the cheese around.) Bake the cheese for 5 minutes, or until the edges of the cheese start to lightly brown. If making the wrap in a regular-size oven or toaster oven, use the same temperature and baking time, being sure to preheat the oven beforehand.

4. Remove the wrap from the air fryer or oven and let cool.

5. Fill the wrap with your favorite sandwich toppings.

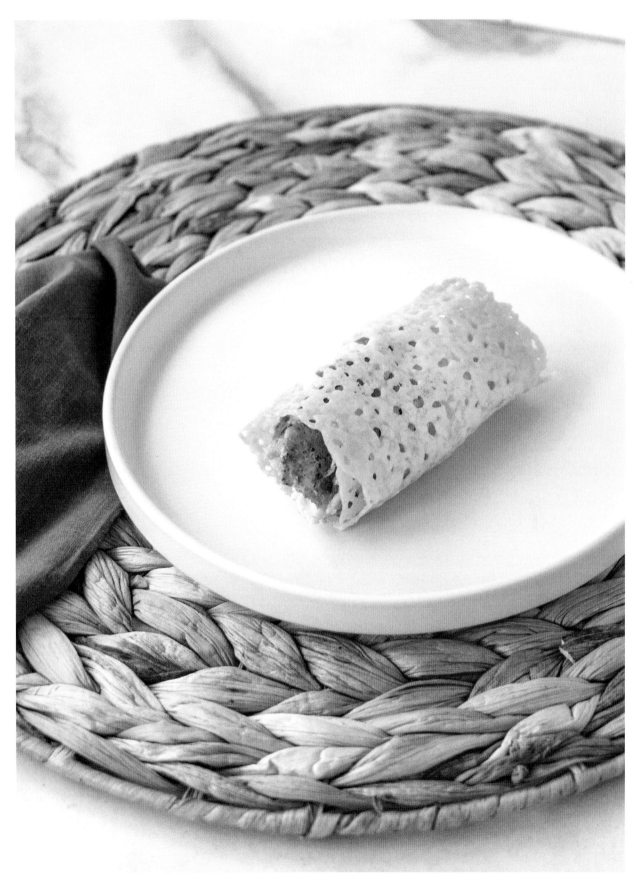

chicken flour

YIELD:
1 cup

PREP TIME:
10 minutes (not including time to cook whole chicken breasts)

COOK TIME:
75 minutes

Chicken flour! You have now officially heard of everything. This is a good option when you're looking for an alternative to pork panko. It isn't an equal swap, though, because chicken flour is very dense; you'll want to use a little more than half of the quantity of pork panko. I use it most often in my doughs for Carnizza (page 182) and "Corn" Dogs (page 188) when I need a non-pork option.

1½ pounds boneless, skinless chicken breasts, cooked (see note)

special equipment:
High-powered blender

1. Preheat the oven to 300°F and line a sheet pan with parchment paper.

2. Cut the cooked chicken into large chunks and place in a food processor. Pulse/chop the chicken to get it into the smallest pieces you can.

3. Spread the chopped chicken on the prepared pan and bake for 60 to 75 minutes, stirring every 20 minutes, until browned and completely dried.

4. After the chicken has cooled, place half of the chicken at a time in a high-powered blender and blend into a fine powder.

Note:

The best method for cooking the chicken is baking (without any added fat), using either a regular oven or air fryer. I threw mine in a preheated air fryer at 400°F for 30 minutes. If using the oven, preheat it to 400°F and bake for 45 to 50 minutes. You want the chicken to be very well cooked, to the point of being dry. Allow the chicken to cool until easy to handle before proceeding with Step 2.

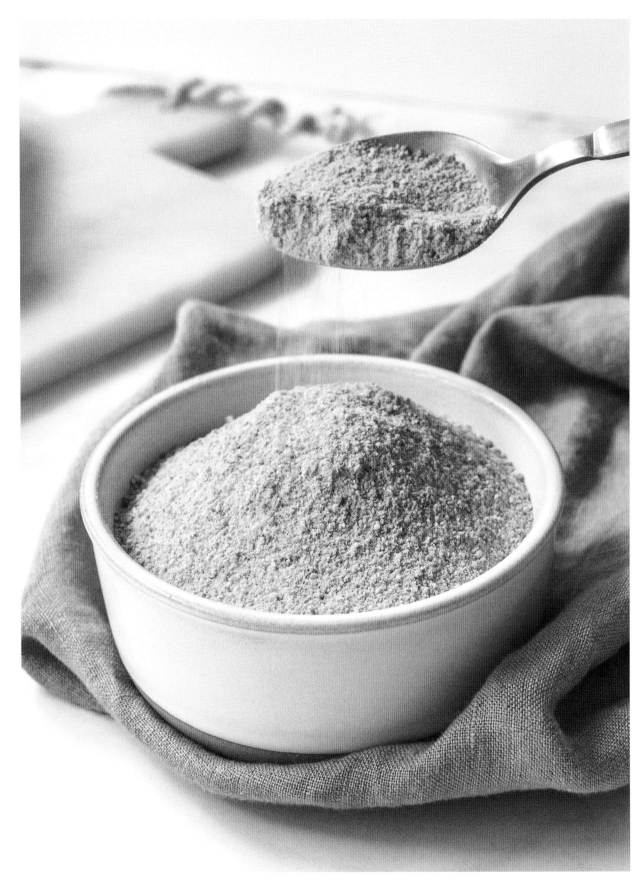

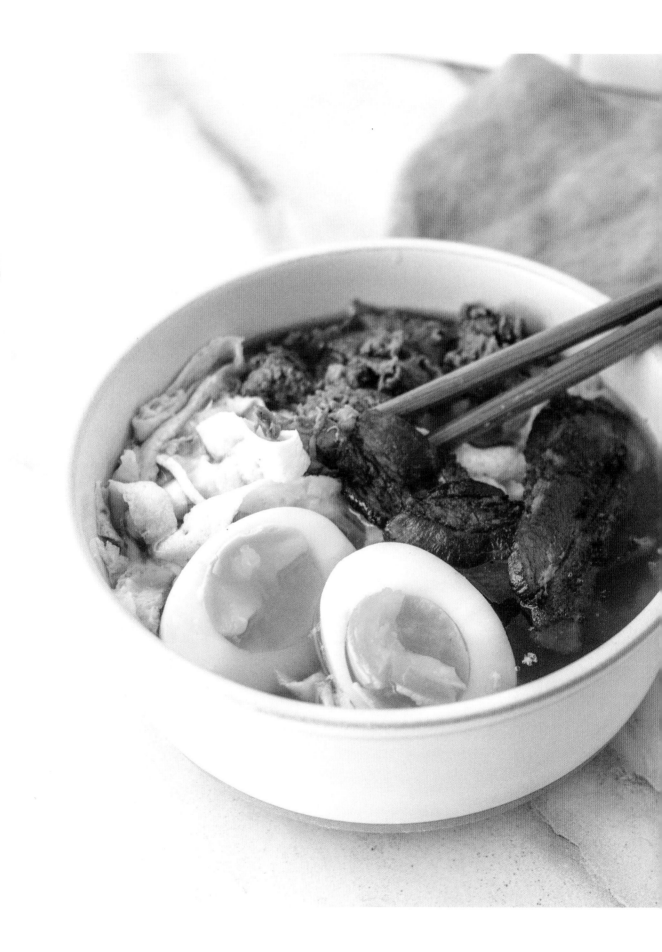

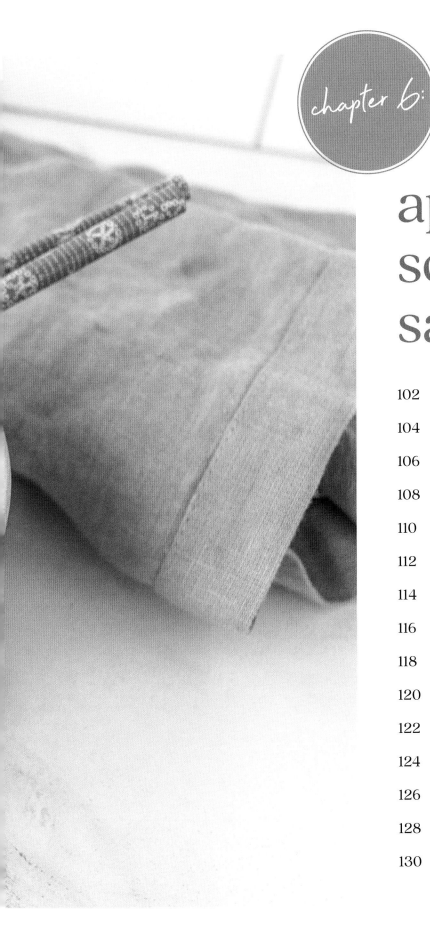

chapter 6:

appetizers, soups & salads

104 • smoked salmon blinis

106 • fried goat cheese balls

108 • meat chips

110 • instant pot deviled eggs

112 • salami cups

114 • fried egg yolks

116 • mozzarella sticks

118 • bacon cheeseburger soup

120 • creamy sausage soup

122 • chicken noodle soup

124 • ramen

126 • sipping bone broth

128 • cobb salad

130 • chicken salad

piggy bites

YIELD:
32 bite-sized pieces
(about 10 servings)

PREP TIME:
20 minutes

COOK TIME:
55 minutes

My community asked for finger foods, so here you are! The texture of these bites is awesome. The bacon is crispy but melts in your mouth. The cheese is soft and warm, and the bottom of the sausage crisps up from the bacon grease. It's quite a party in your mouth. These are great to assemble ahead of time and bake before serving.

1 pound regular, thin-cut bacon (about 16 slices)

10 ounces fully cooked smoked sausage

5 ounces (10 tablespoons) cream cheese

5 ounces fresh (soft) goat cheese

1. Preheat the oven to 400°F. Line a sheet pan with parchment paper.

2. Cut the bacon slices in half crosswise to make about 32 pieces, depending on the number of bacon slices in your package of bacon.

3. Slice the sausage crosswise into roughly 32 discs, to match the number of bacon pieces.

4. Take a piece of sausage and wrap the bacon around it, making something that resembles a little shot glass. The sausage is the bottom of the shot glass, while the bacon acts as the sides. Secure the bacon to the sausage with a toothpick, running it horizontally through the sausage, so that the toothpick is positioned parallel to the sausage.

5. Mix the 2 cheeses and microwave for 30 seconds to warm it so it's soft.

6. Add the cheese to a zip-top plastic bag and cut a bottom corner from the bag to use it as a piping bag.

7. Pipe the cheese into the little piggy shot glasses, filling them nearly to the top. If you overfill them, the cheese mixture will run over during baking.

8. Place all the pieces onto the prepared pan.

9. Bake until the bacon is crispy, 45 to 55 minutes.

10. Serve warm, but they are delicious as cold leftovers too.

Note:

Regular, thin-cut bacon is ideal; thick-cut bacon is too thick to wrap properly. I recommend kielbasa for this recipe, but any smoked, fully cooked sausage should do great.

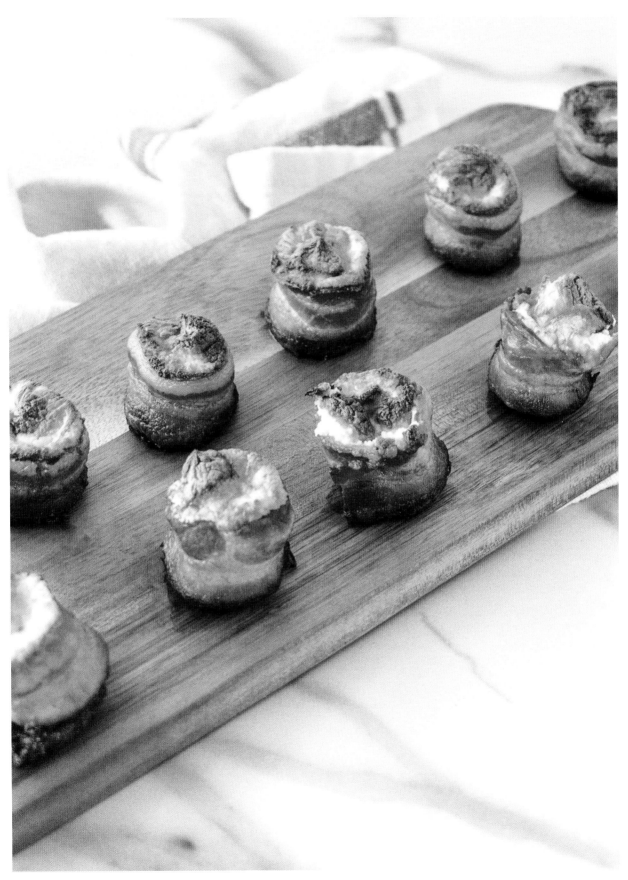

smoked salmon blinis

YIELD:
10 bite-size blinis
(3 to 4 servings)

PREP TIME:
15 minutes (not including
time to make batter)

COOK TIME:
8 minutes

If you're looking to impress guests or you just want to switch up your eggs-and-bacon breakfast routine, put these blinis on the menu. They are perfect for brunch or as a fancy cocktail appetizer. And although they look elegant, they're super simple to make. Of course, the sprig of dill isn't carnivore, but it's so pretty and pairs nicely with salmon, so I love to use it.

2 tablespoons salted butter, divided, for the pan

½ batch All-Purpose Waffle batter (page 86)

5 ounces (10 tablespoons) cream cheese, softened

4 ounces cold-smoked salmon

Fresh dill sprig, snipped into 10 small pieces, for garnish (optional)

1. Preheat a medium-size skillet over medium heat until hot but not yet smoking.

2. Drop half of the butter into the hot skillet. Once the butter is melted, drop 1 tablespoon of the batter into the pan and, using the back of a spoon, spread the batter out to make a small pancake, about 2 inches in diameter. Repeat four more times to cook a total of five pancakes at once, using about half of the batter.

3. Cook the pancakes until browned, about 2 minutes, then flip and cook for 2 more minutes, or until browned on both sides. Remove to a plate to cool.

4. Repeat with the remaining butter and batter to make five more pancakes.

5. Once cool, top each blini with 1 tablespoon of cream cheese. I like to put the cream cheese in a plastic baggie and cut off one corner so it can be piped on nicely.

6. Gently top each blini with a small piece of smoked salmon, folded to fit and look pretty.

7. Garnish each blini with a tiny piece of fresh dill, if desired.

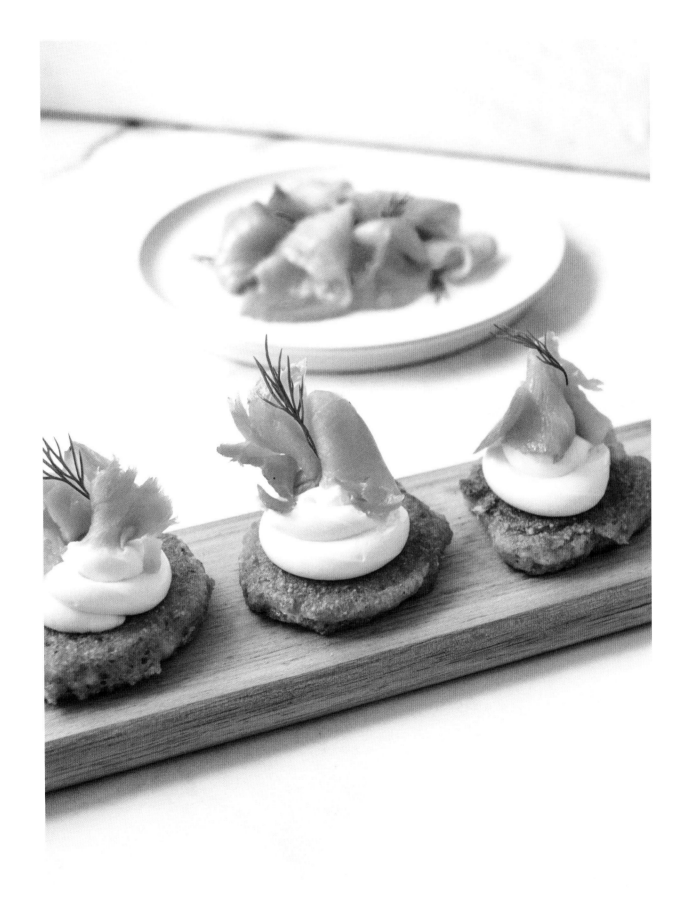

fried goat cheese balls

YIELD:
8 (2-inch) balls (4 servings)

PREP TIME:
15 minutes

COOK TIME:
8 minutes

I love to make these delightful little things when I have company; they're always a huge hit. If you're entertaining a larger group, you can easily double the recipe. When you're coating these, I recommend using one hand for the panko and the other for the egg. This prevents your hands from getting messy and keeps the egg from making the panko soggy. I like to work in two batches using a medium-size pot, but if you're going to make a lot, feel free to use a large pan. Just make sure you have a nice layer of fat to fry them in.

1 cup pork panko, divided

1 large egg

1 (10.5-ounce) log fresh (soft) goat cheese

¼ cup tallow or other heat-tolerant fat of choice, plus extra if needed, for frying

1. Prepare a coating station: Set 3 small bowls in a row. Put ¼ cup of the pork panko in the first bowl on the left, and put the remaining ¾ cup of panko in the third bowl on the right. Crack the egg into the middle bowl and whisk well.

2. Divide the goat cheese into 8 equal pieces and roll each piece into a ball.

3. Dip a ball into the first bowl of panko and roll to give it a light dusting, which will help the egg stick. Place the ball in the bowl of egg, coating well, then place in the third bowl and completely cover the ball with panko. Set aside on a plate.

4. Repeat with the remaining balls.

5. Place the plate of coated balls in the freezer while you heat the oil. This ensures that the cheese will not ooze out when cooking. You want the center of the cheese balls to get hot, so don't leave them in the freezer for more than 10 minutes.

6. To heat the oil, put the tallow in a deep-sided skillet or shallow saucepot or Dutch oven that's 8 to 10 inches in diameter and set over medium-high heat. Make sure you have about ¼ inch of melted tallow; add more tallow if needed. You'll know the fat is hot enough when you put a pinch of panko in the tallow and it sizzles.

7. Set 4 of the balls in the hot fat and cook for 3 to 4 minutes, turning frequently, until the entire surface of the balls becomes brown. It is important to cook quickly with hot oil or the cheese can ooze out.

8. Transfer the balls to a paper towel–lined plate to drain.

9. Repeat with the remaining balls, adding more tallow as necessary to keep the depth consistent. Serve immediately.

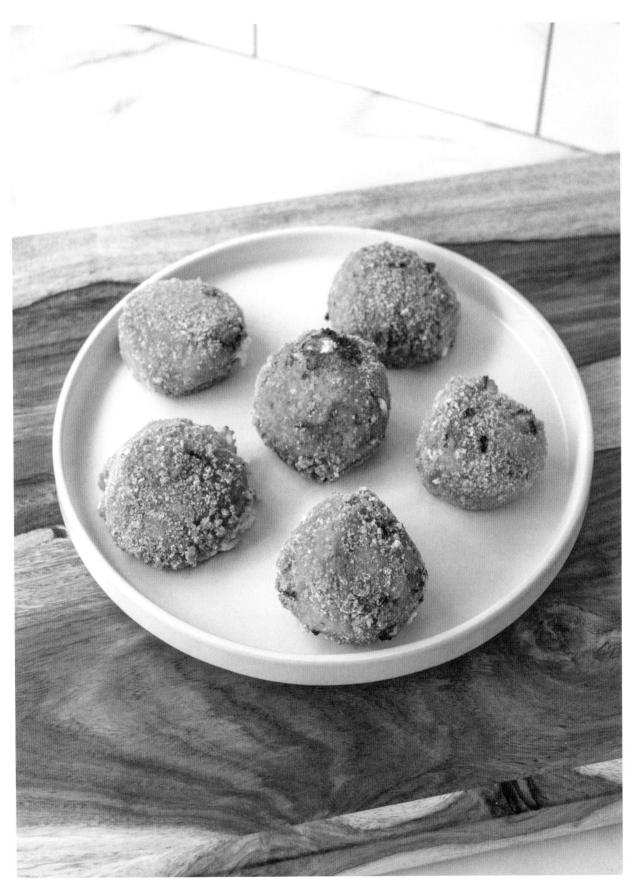

meat chips

YIELD:
4 servings

PREP TIME:
20 minutes

COOK TIME:
10 to 14 hours

These are by far one of my favorite things to eat—and my kids' too. When I make them, we immediately devour the entire batch. I don't even wait for them to cool down. Having them warm, with their flaky texture and saltiness, is pure heaven. When slicing the meat, I recommend cutting it into 3-mm-thick rounds for a dippable chip. I also like to cut it even thinner—just 2 mm thick—which makes for a wafer-thin and delicate chip, but then they're too fragile for dipping. My mouth is watering just talking about these! This recipe requires a food dehydrator and an electric meat slicer. If you don't already own these, I hope my description of these chips convinces you to get them. It's worth it!

1 (1-pound) tube ground beef, frozen (do not defrost)

Kosher salt

Whipped Goat Cheese Dip (page 214) or other dip of choice, for serving (optional)

1. Using an electric meat slicer, cut the frozen ground beef into 3-mm- or 2-mm-thick rounds. They will curl a bit as they are cut, but no worries; simply unroll and place on the food dehydrator racks. Sprinkle the chips lightly with salt.

2. If you've cut the meat into to 3-mm chips, cook it at 165°F for 12 to 14 hours, depending on your preferred texture. If you've cut it into 2-mm chips, cook it at 165°F for 10 hours.

3. Serve with your favorite dip, if desired.

special equipment:
Electric meat slicer and food dehydrator

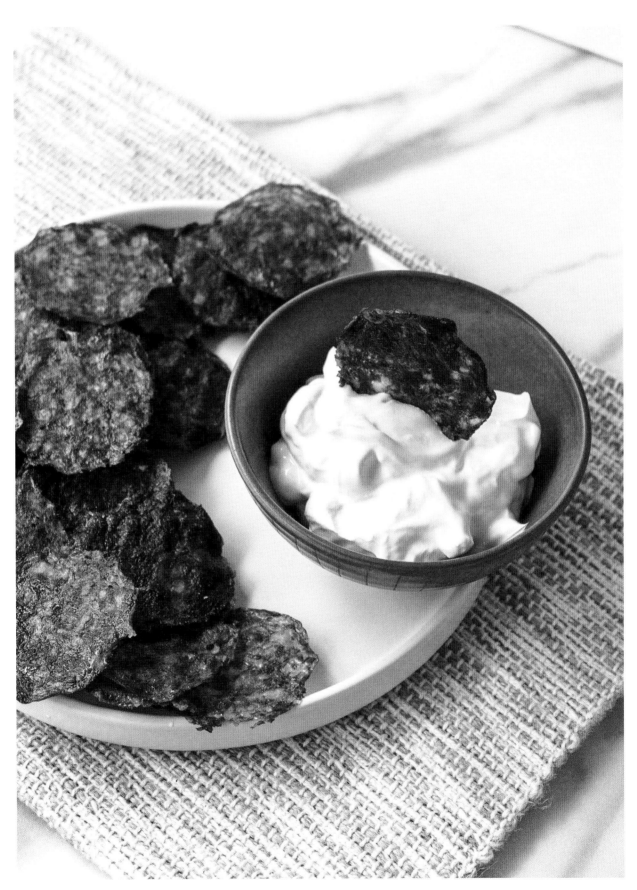

instant pot deviled eggs

YIELD:
12 deviled eggs (4 servings)

PREP TIME:
20 minutes (not including time to make mayo)

COOK TIME:
5 minutes

Don't save fun foods for when you have guests over. Add these to your meal prep list! They are great to grab on a busy morning as you're heading out the door. Instead of hard-cooking the eggs in boiling water, I like to steam them in an Instant Pot, which makes them very easy to peel. Of course, you can always go the traditional boiling route if you prefer. I recommend using my Butter Bacon Mayonnaise for this recipe, but feel free to use store-bought. If you do, I suggest buying one that uses either avocado oil or coconut oil. Be sure to read ingredient lists because some front labels say avocado oil and then include vegetable oil as well.

6 large eggs

3 tablespoons Butter Bacon Mayonnaise (page 210)

Kosher salt

Chopped cooked bacon, for garnish (optional)

1. Place 6 eggs on a trivet in an Instant Pot.

2. Add ½ cup of water, secure the lid, and select pressure cook on high heat for 5 minutes.

3. When the cook time is up, immediately flip the valve to quickly release all the pressure.

4. As soon as all the pressure has been released and you are able to open the lid, remove the eggs from the Instant Pot and place them in an ice bath until completely cool, 5 to 10 minutes.

5. Peel the eggs, then cut them in half lengthwise. Pop out the yolks and place the yolks in a small bowl or a mini food processor.

6. Add the mayo to the yolks and blend. Add salt to taste.

7. Fill the whites with the yolk mixture, either with a spoon or by piping it in using a plastic baggie with a corner cut off.

8. Top with chopped bacon, if you'd like.

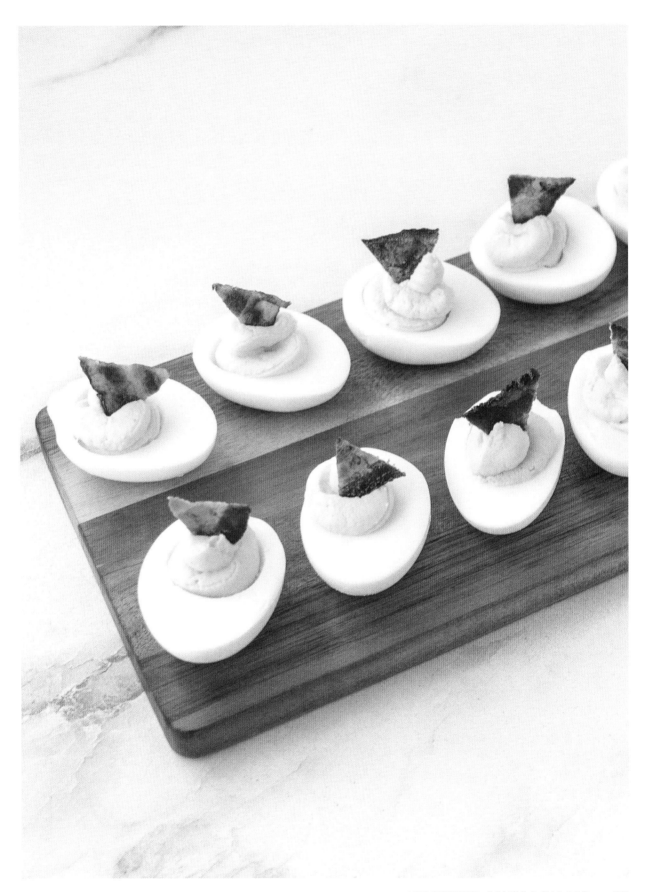

salami cups

YIELD:
24 salami cups (8 servings)

PREP TIME:
10 minutes

COOK TIME:
8 minutes

Back in my boat cheffing days, I used to make these little guys for a family on their yacht, which was based in the San Juan Islands for the summer. These delicious bites were the perfect appetizer to enjoy at cocktail hour with friends on the top deck. But these aren't exclusive to yachts. Standing in your kitchen and eating them off your cutting board is just fine too. These vessels are great for putting whatever you like in them! The recipe calls for feta cheese, but goat cheese, cream cheese, or even olive tapenade (for my animal-based friends) are also good options.

24 slices Italian dry salami (about 4 ounces) (see note)

4 ounces feta cheese, crumbled (about 1 cup)

1. Preheat the oven to 400°F.

2. Line each cup of a 24-well nonstick mini muffin pan with a salami slice, pressing the slices into the bottom and sides of the cups.

3. Bake until crunchy and browned, about 8 minutes. Keep an eye on them so they don't burn.

4. Let cool for a few minutes in the pan before removing. Fill the salami cups with pieces of feta and serve. Serve leftovers chilled or at room temperature.

Note:

The salami I use is precut, Italian dry; the slices are about 2½ inches in diameter and 2 mm thick.

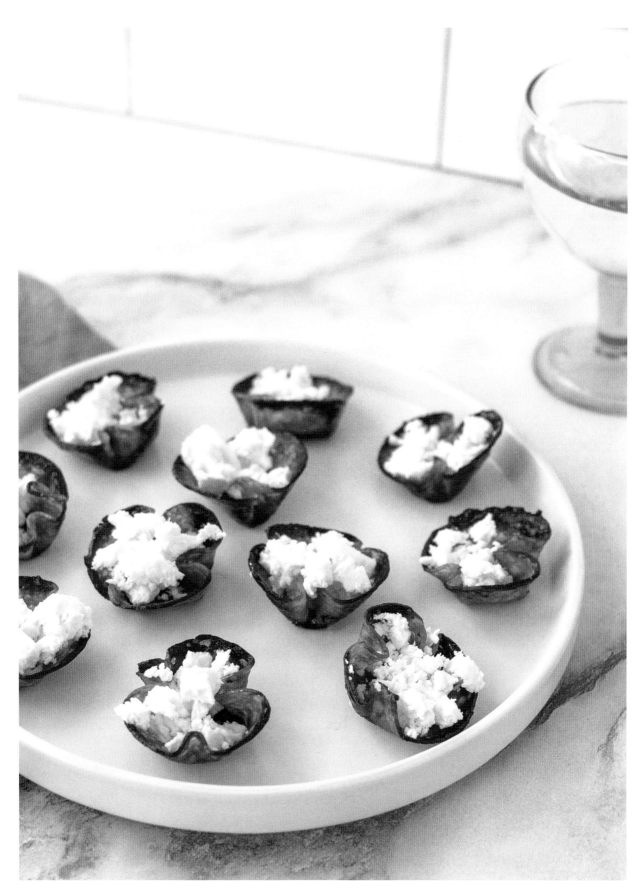

fried egg yolks

YIELD:
2 to 4 servings

PREP TIME:
10 minutes

COOK TIME:
2 to 4 minutes, depending on preferred doneness

When cooking these, I keep them on the runnier side for topping burgers but cook them until set if I'm eating them by themselves as finger food. If you're serving these to guests, you may want to do the latter so there aren't any surprises with yolk oozing out.

¼ cup pork panko

5 large eggs

1 tablespoon bacon grease or fat of choice, for the pan

Pinch of kosher salt, for garnish

1. Put the panko in a medium-size bowl.

2. Gently separate the yolks from the whites (see note), then gently set the yolks on top of the panko.

3. Lightly move the yolks around to cover all the surfaces in panko; be careful not to break them.

4. Preheat a medium-size skillet over medium-high heat, then add the cooking fat and swirl to coat.

5. Cook for about 2 minutes on each side for hard-cooked yolks. They will be firm to the touch when done. For a slightly runny yolk, cook for about 1 minute on each side. They will still feel squishy when done.

6. Top with a sprinkle of salt. Serve immediately.

Note: *Be sure to save the whites to make wraps or noodles (see page 94).*

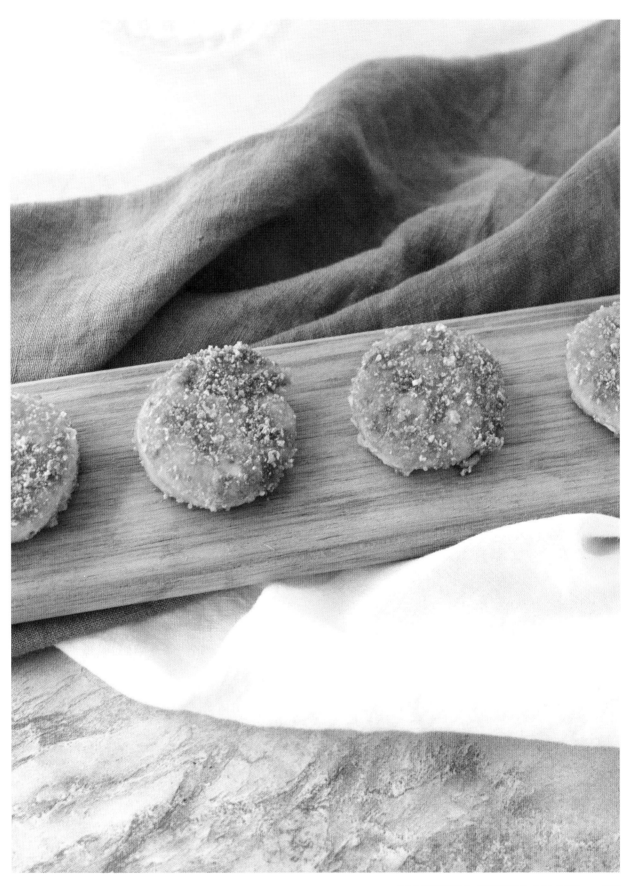

mozzarella sticks

YIELD:
6 sticks (2 servings)

PREP TIME:
5 minutes, plus 20 minutes
to chill

COOK TIME:
4 minutes

Want to eat several cold, rubbery string cheeses at once? No thanks. Want to eat string cheeses that have been coated in panko and deep-fried until golden and crispy with a molten interior? Heck yes! These crispy, cheesy sticks of heaven are a perfect snack or party appetizer. Back in my bar-hopping days, they were a must-order. Now, my days are a little less alcohol filled, but I still love this old favorite bar food. We snack on them just as they are, but if you're a rebel, you can dip them in marinara sauce. I won't tell.

¼ cup plus 2 tablespoons pork panko, divided

1 large egg

3 whole-milk mozzarella string cheese sticks, cut in half crosswise (see notes)

½ cup tallow, bacon grease, or other heat-tolerant fat of choice, plus extra if needed, for frying

Dipping sauce of choice, for serving (optional)

1. Prepare a coating station: Set 3 small bowls in a row. Put 2 tablespoons of the pork panko in the first bowl on the left, and then put the remaining ¼ cup of panko in the third bowl on the right. Crack the egg into the middle bowl and whisk well.

2. Take a cheese stick and press it into the first bowl of panko, coating all sides; this will help the egg stick better.

3. Dip the stick into the egg, then press it into the last bowl of panko, again coating all sides. Set all the coated pieces on a plate and pop it in the freezer for 20 minutes. This ensures that the cheese will hold up to frying and won't leak through the breading.

4. After the sticks have chilled for 15 minutes, heat the tallow in a deep-sided skillet or a shallow sauce pot or Dutch oven that's 8 to 10 inches in diameter over medium-high heat until it reaches 350°F. Make sure you have about ½ inch of melted tallow; add more tallow if needed.

5. Fry the in the hot fat for 3 to 4 minutes, flipping them around every minute to ensure all sides get browned and crispy. When done, remove the sticks to a paper towel–lined plate to drain.

6. Serve immediately. Eat as is or serve with your favorite dipping sauce.

Notes:

While the carnivore diet prioritizes full-fat dairy, part-skim cheese sticks can be used here.

Just like in the recipe for Fried Goat Cheese Balls (page 106), when coating the cheese sticks, I suggest you use one hand for the panko and the other for the egg. That will help prevent your hands from getting too messy and keep the egg from making the panko soggy.

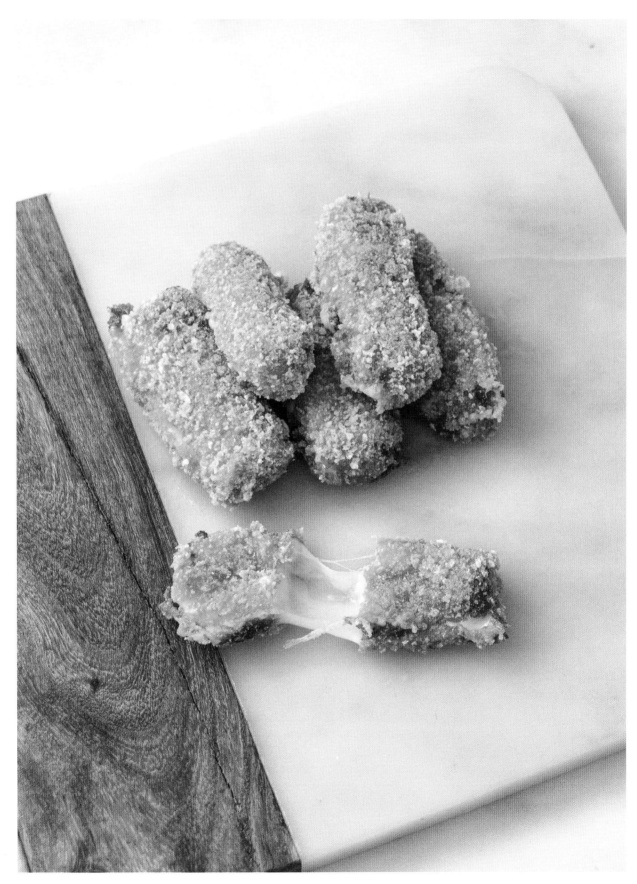

bacon cheeseburger soup

YIELD:
2 to 4 servings

PREP TIME:
10 minutes (not including time to cook bacon)

COOK TIME:
20 minutes

This recipe is extra special to me because it was the first one I shared with my private Facebook community for feedback. It received rave reviews, and I hope you love it too. I highly recommend you make a double batch to help with meal prep for the week. It reheats well, and your future self will thank you for making enough for leftovers. If you include some fruit in your diet, chopped pickles would be a delicious topping to add before serving.

1 tablespoon tallow or other heat-tolerant fat of choice, for the pot

1 pound ground beef

1 cup beef broth, homemade (page 126) or store-bought

4 ounces (½ cup) cream cheese

½ cup heavy cream

2 cups shredded cheddar cheese (about 8 ounces)

Kosher salt

FOR GARNISH:

6 slices regular, thin-cut bacon, cooked (see page 166) and coarsely chopped

½ to ¾ cup shredded cheddar cheese (2 to 3 ounces)

1. Preheat a medium-size Dutch oven or similarly sized soup pot over medium-high heat. When hot, drop in the tallow and swirl to coat the pot. Add the ground beef and cook the meat, while stirring to break it apart, until browned and cooked through, about 15 minutes. Drain the fat.

2. Add the broth, cream cheese, and heavy cream.

3. Bring the soup to a low simmer, still over medium-high heat, while stirring occasionally to blend in the cream cheese, about 5 minutes.

4. Once the soup is simmering, turn off the heat, add the cheddar cheese, and stir until well combined.

5. Salt the soup to taste. You may find it won't need much or any at all, depending on the salt content of the broth. Keep in mind that the bacon garnish will add saltiness as well.

6. Serve immediately, garnished with the chopped bacon and shredded cheese.

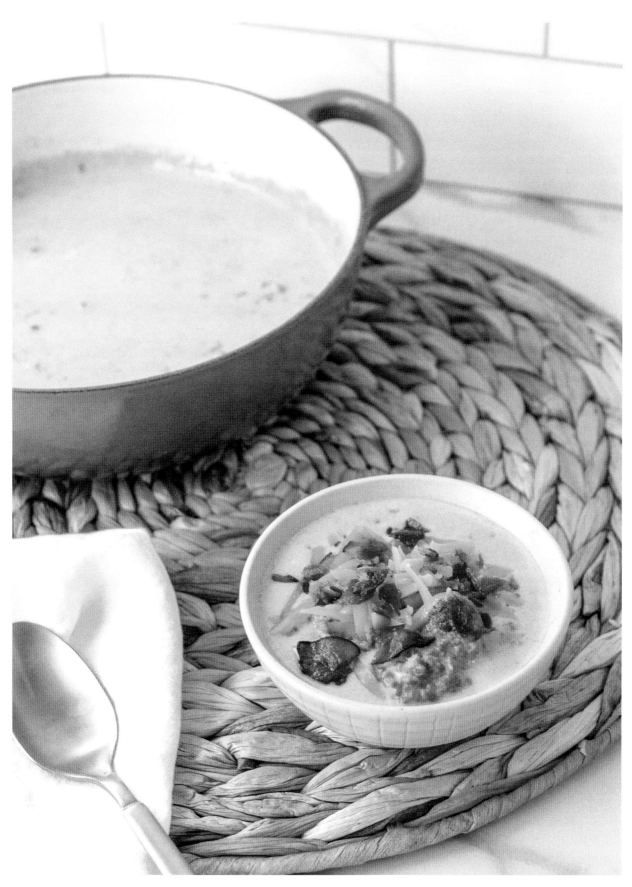

creamy sausage soup

YIELD:
2 to 4 servings

PREP TIME:
5 minutes

COOK TIME:
20 minutes

I made a version of this recipe early in my carnivore days, and it went viral, with the internet dubbing it "Meat Cereal." (There was even an article written about it on food.ndtv.com.) I've got to say, that description isn't wrong. It does kind of look like a bowl of cereal. But the joke's on the critics, because this soup is so delicious. It is great for batch cooking and having a ready-to-heat meal in the refrigerator. I hope you love to eat it as much as the internet loved to mock it!

1 tablespoon tallow or other heat-tolerant fat of choice, for the pot

1 pound bulk sausage of choice

1 cup beef broth, homemade (page 126) or store-bought

1 (8-ounce) package cream cheese

Kosher salt

1. Preheat a medium-size Dutch oven or similarly sized soup pot over medium-high heat until hot and just beginning to smoke. Drop in the tallow and swirl to coat the pot.

2. Add the sausage and cook, stirring to break it into small pieces, until browned and cooked through, about 10 minutes. Drain all but 2 tablespoons of the fat.

3. Add the broth and cream cheese to the sausage.

4. Simmer over medium heat, stirring occasionally, until the cream cheese is melted and the soup is hot, about 10 minutes.

5. Salt the soup to taste; it may not need much if any, depending on the amount of salt in the sausage and broth.

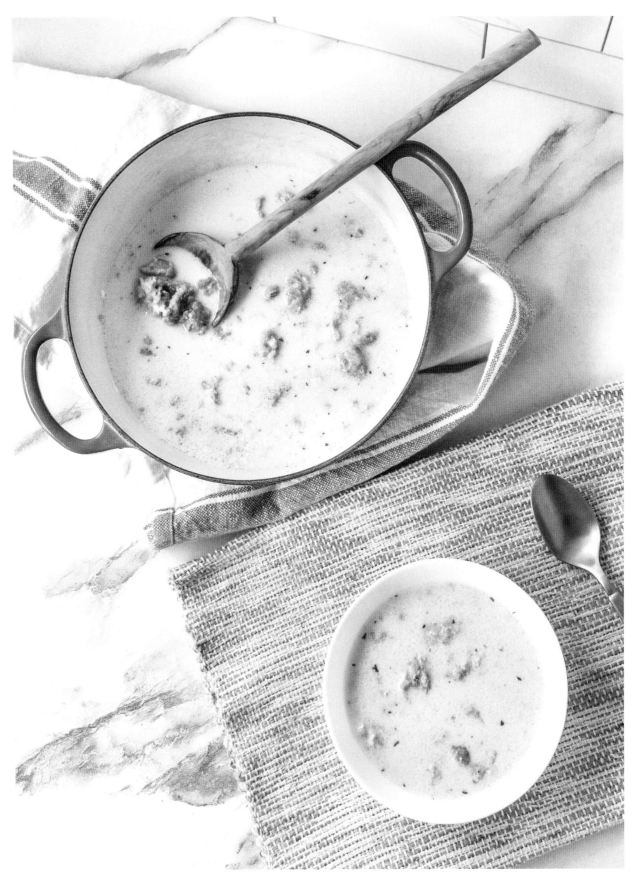

chicken noodle soup

YIELD:
2 servings

PREP TIME:
5 minutes (not including time to cook chicken or noodles)

COOK TIME:
10 minutes

I must give my husband credit for this recipe. It's the collaboration he never wanted. I make a carnivore egg drop soup (which is just broth and eggs) all the time, but one night he suggested I add my noodles and some chicken to make a chicken noodle soup. Eggs in a chicken noodle soup is so yummy that you won't even miss the carrots and celery. This reheats nicely, so make a double batch if you want lunch ready for the week.

4 cups chicken broth, homemade (page 126) or store-bought

4 large eggs, whisked

8 ounces cooked, chopped chicken (dark meat)

1 batch Egg White Noodles (page 94)

Kosher salt

1. In a medium-size Dutch oven or similarly sized soup pot, bring the broth to a low boil over medium-high heat.

2. Turn the heat down to low and slowly drizzle in the eggs while whisking.

3. Add the cooked chicken and noodles and allow them to heat up for a minute.

4. Turn off the heat, add salt to taste, and serve immediately.

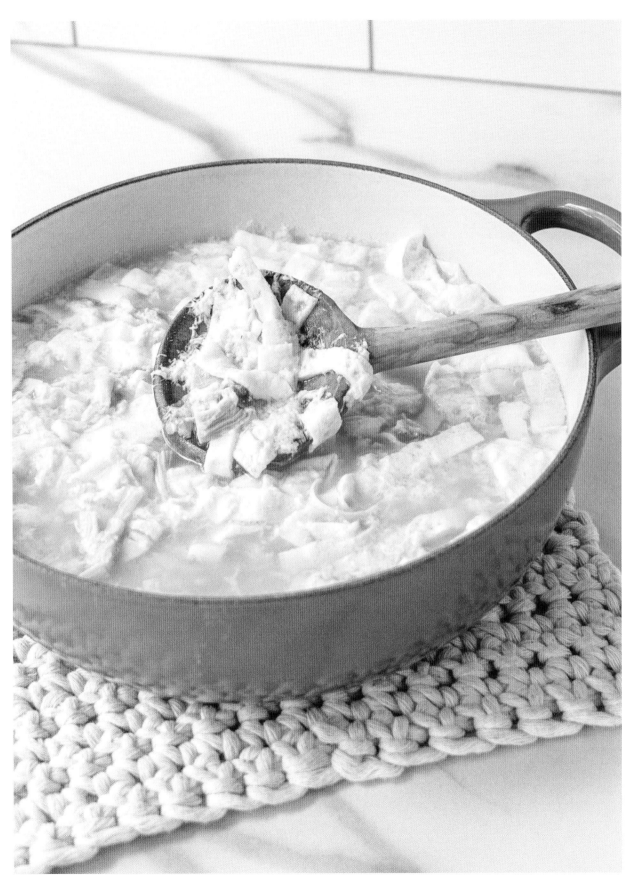

ramen

YIELD:
2 servings

PREP TIME:
5 minutes (not including time to cook noodles, bacon, or eggs)

COOK TIME:
15 minutes

Ramen is a hearty, feel-good, comforting meal. It's also versatile, so feel free to use any meats and toppings you love; here, I have included my favorites. For meal prep, double or triple the ingredients, store the prepared components separately, and assemble the bowls just before serving.

4 cups chicken or beef broth, homemade (page 126) or store-bought

1 tablespoon tallow or other heat-tolerant fat of choice, for the pot

½ pound shaved beef (see notes)

Double batch Egg White Noodles (page 94)

4 slices regular, thin-cut bacon, cooked (see page 166) and cut in half crosswise

2 large medium-cooked eggs (see notes), peeled and cut in half

1. In a medium-size Dutch oven or similarly sized soup pot, bring the broth to a simmer over high heat.

2. Meanwhile, preheat a medium skillet over medium-high heat until just beginning to smoke. Drop in the tallow and swirl to coat the pan. Add the shaved beef and cook for about 2 minutes on each side, until cooked through.

3. To serve, divide the hot broth between 2 large soup bowls. To each bowl, add half of the noodles, half of the shaved beef, 4 pieces of bacon, and 2 egg halves.

 Notes:

Shaved beef is very thinly sliced beef, or steak, that is most often intended for a hot pot. I buy it precut. You can ask a butcher to cut it for you; request that a boneless sirloin steak be sliced paper thin. You also can use a meat slicer at home.

The ideal texture of the egg yolks for this recipe is just set: they should no longer be runny, but the yolk should be very creamy. To make medium-cooked eggs, use the Instant Pot method described in the Instant Pot Deviled Eggs recipe on page 110, reducing the cooking time to 2 minutes.

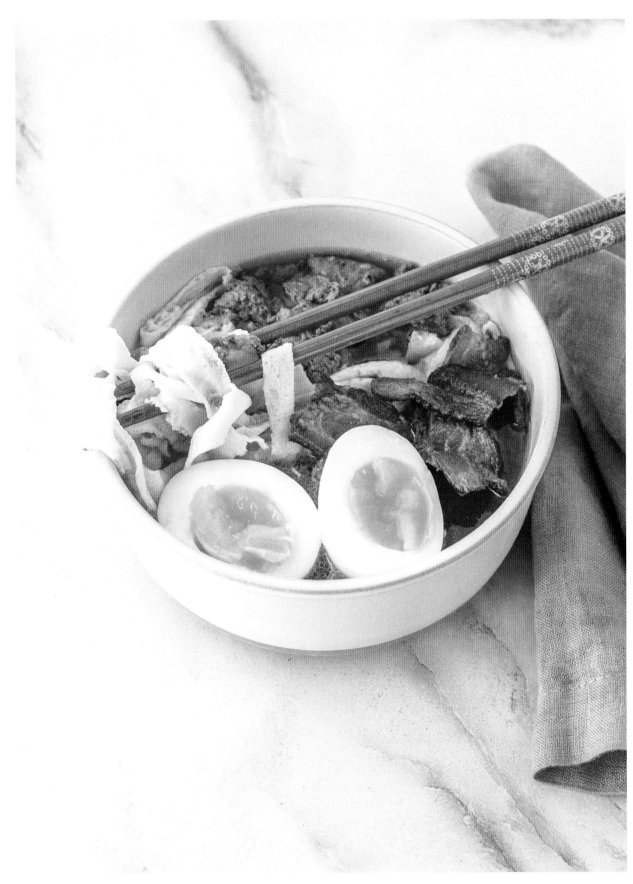

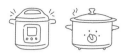

sipping bone broth

YIELD:
8 cups (8 servings)

PREP TIME:
5 minutes

COOK TIME:
3 or 12 hours, depending on method

Whenever you cook bone-in cuts of meat, freeze the bones in a zip-top plastic bag so you can use them to make broth later. Some stores sell bones for making broth; marrow bones are especially nice (eat the marrow!), as are chicken feet. Both will make your broth rich and gelatinous. Flavorwise, marrow bones are ideally suited to beef broth, and chicken feet to—you guessed it—chicken broth. But I often use chicken feet for beef broth and vice versa, depending on what I have on hand. You can also mix up the types of bones (for example, chicken feet, neck, leg, and back) or use a mix of bones from different animals (for example, beef and chicken). Sip on this broth in the morning, or add it to soups and stews, such as Bacon Cheeseburger Soup (page 118). I salt the prepared broth as I use it, especially when sipping on it, instead of when making it. If you have extra broth, I recommend pouring it into silicone molds or an ice cube tray and freezing it; once frozen, pop the cubes into a freezer bag and store in the freezer for whenever you need broth. You can make this in either an Instant Pot or a slow cooker.

3 pounds beef or chicken bones, or a combination of both

8 ounces marrow bones (see note) or chicken feet (about 6)

Filtered water (about 8 cups)

Kosher salt (optional)

1. Put the bones in an Instant Pot or slow cooker and fill with filtered water until just covered, about 8 cups. If using a slow cooker, skip ahead to Step 3.

2. If using an Instant Pot, secure the lid and set to pressure cook on high for 3 hours. Once finished, quick-release the pressure. Skip ahead to Step 4.

3. If using a slow cooker, cook on low heat for a minimum of 12 hours and as long as 24 hours.

4. Strain the broth, discarding the bones. You can remove the fat, if you like, using a fat separator. If you don't have a fat separator, simply put the cooled broth in the refrigerator; once chilled, the fat will form a solid layer on the top, and you can remove it. Also note that the marrow bones or chicken feet will make this broth very gelatinous. It will look like Jell-O in the refrigerator but will liquefy when rewarmed.

5. Keep the broth in a sealed glass jar or pitcher in the refrigerator for up to 5 days or freeze any extra. If desired, season the broth with salt to taste before using.

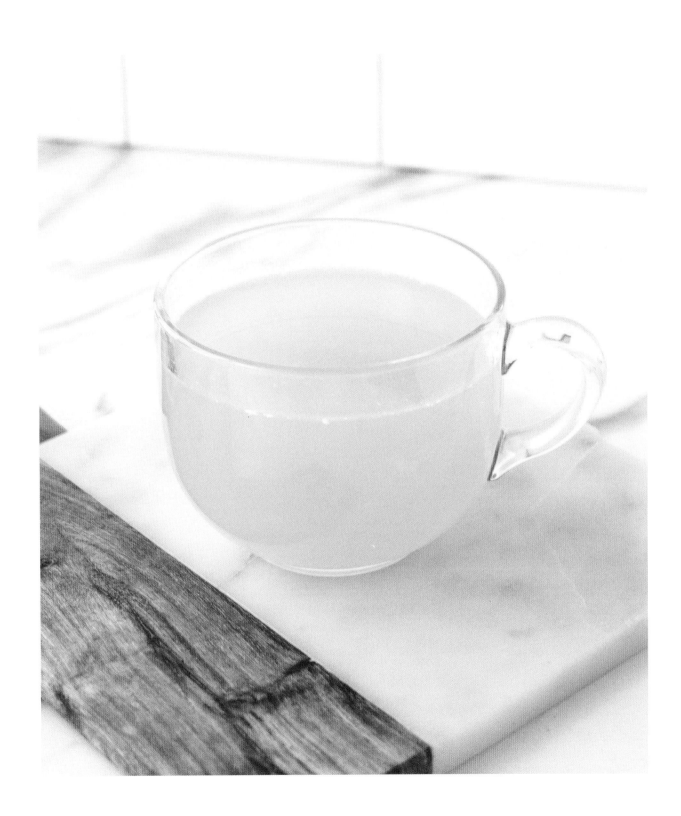

Note: If using marrow bones, have your butcher cut them into about 4-inch lengths. The exact size doesn't matter, just so the pieces are small enough to fit into your pot.

cobb salad

YIELD:
4 servings

PREP TIME:
15 minutes (not including time
to cook chicken, bacon, and eggs)

As much as I love my steaks, I did enjoy eating salads in my pre-carnivore days—although, if I'm being honest, I mainly liked the meats, cheeses, and dressings. This carnivore salad hits the spot, and while it doesn't have any lettuce, if you wanted to add some, it wouldn't be the end of the world. If you have any leftover dressing, you can store it in the refrigerator, but know that it will solidify; simply warm it a tad so you can drizzle it over the salad.

1 batch Pan-Seared
Chicken Breast (page 146),
sliced

½ pound regular, thin-cut
bacon, cooked (see page
166) and coarsely chopped

4 large hard-cooked eggs
(see note), peeled and
halved

½ cup crumbled
Gorgonzola cheese (about
2 ounces)

FOR THE DRESSING:

⅓ cup salted butter,
melted

2 tablespoons Dijon
mustard

1. Assemble the meats, eggs, and cheese on 4 salad plates.

2. To make the dressing, blend the ingredients in a mini food processor, or put the ingredients in a lidded bottle or mason jar and shake vigorously.

3. Drizzle the dressing over the salad and enjoy.

 To cook the eggs, I recommend using the cooking method in the recipe for Instant Pot Deviled Eggs (page 110).

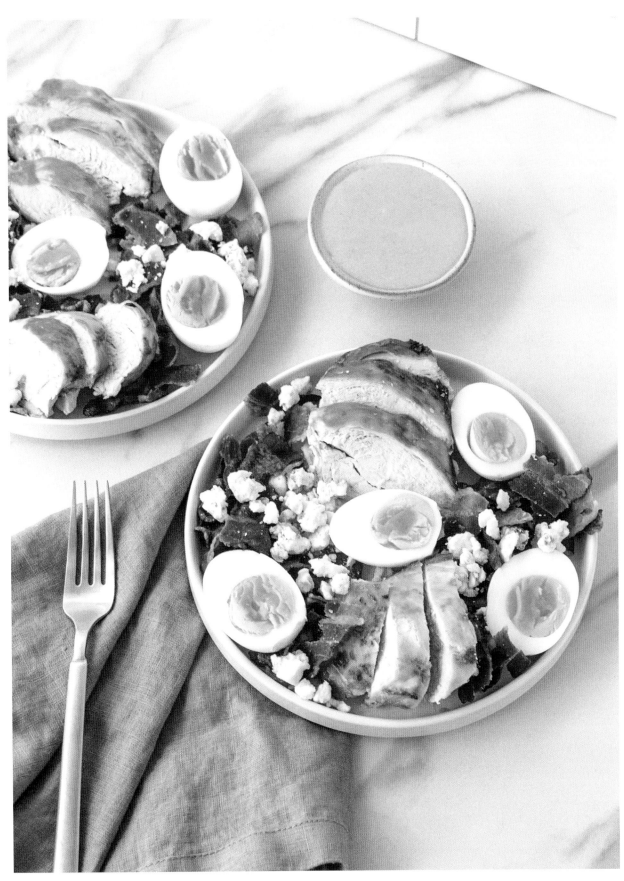

chicken salad

YIELD:
2 servings

PREP TIME:
10 minutes (not including time to make chicken, mayo, or bacon)

I love making a double batch of this salad for easy lunches for the week. You can cook the chicken however you like; pan-searing it using the recipe on page 146 is always a good option. The kiddos enjoy this salad and often eat it with Meat Chips (page 108) or pork rinds for scooping!

1 pound boneless, skinless chicken breast, cooked

½ cup Butter Bacon Mayonnaise (page 210)

3 slices regular, thin-cut bacon, cooked (see page 166) and chopped

Kosher salt

1. Chop the chicken into small pieces and put in a medium-size bowl.

2. Add the mayo to the chicken and mix well.

3. Stir in the bacon. Add salt to taste—you may need only a tiny amount.

4. Serve chilled.

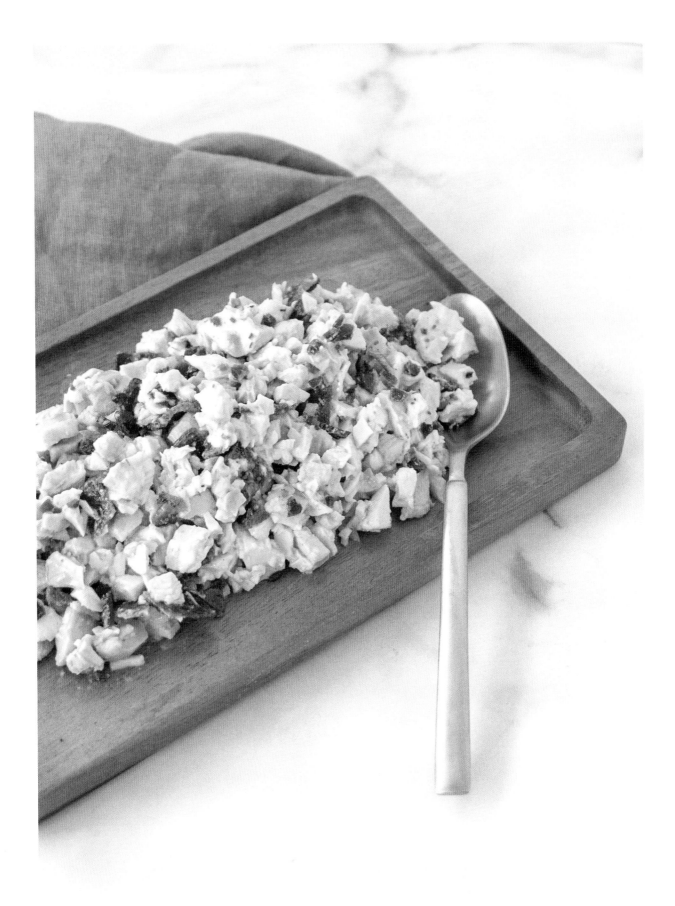

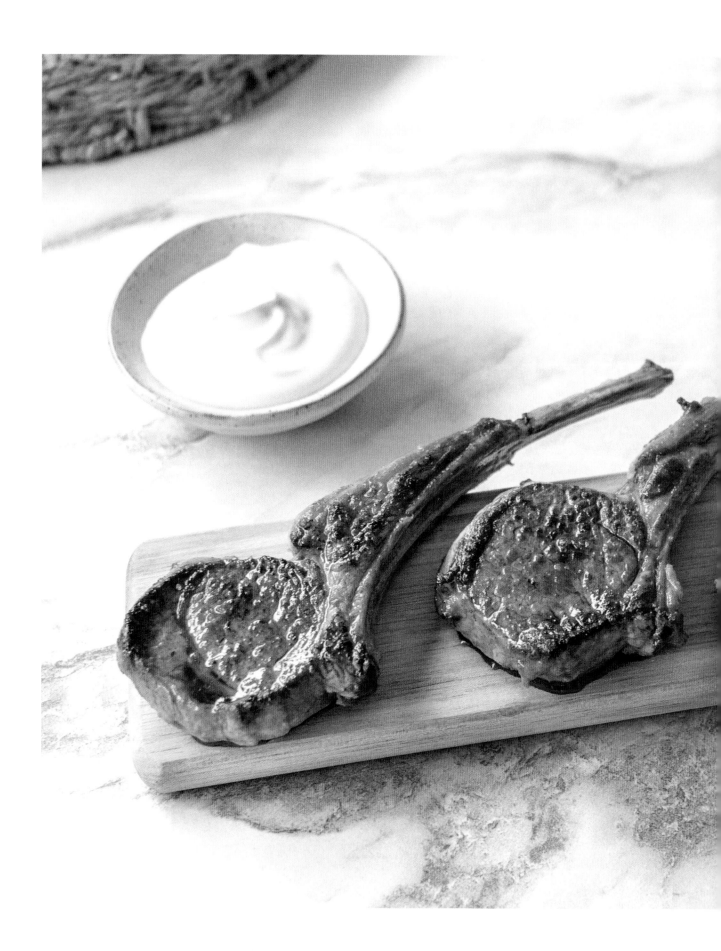

chapter 7:

simply meat

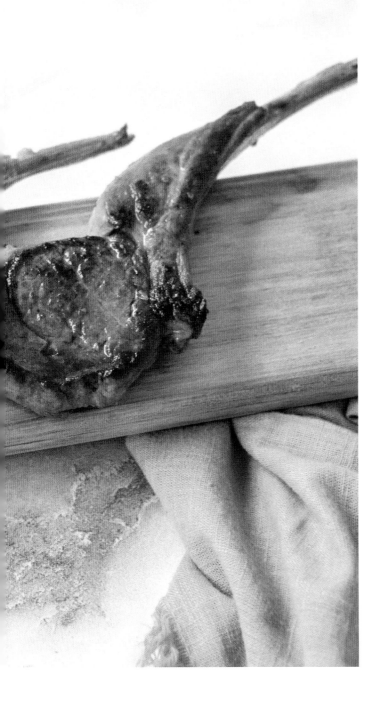

filet mignon

YIELD:
2 servings

PREP TIME:
5 minutes

COOK TIME:
14 to 18 minutes, depending on preferred doneness

Filet mignon is a fabulous cut of steak. It is lean but oh-so-tender. I prefer a combo pan-sear plus oven cooking method when steaks are really thick like these. It allows the interior to cook perfectly without burning the exterior. These filets are great when you have guests over because they have a fancy vibe to them and make a nice plating presentation. Serve them as is or topped with a sauce, such as Blue Cheese Cream Sauce (page 216), or simply a pat of butter.

2 (8-ounce) filet mignons, about 1½ inches thick

Kosher salt

1 tablespoon tallow or other heat-tolerant fat of choice, for the pan

1. Preheat the oven to 400°F.

2. Preheat a medium-size cast-iron skillet or other oven-safe pan over medium-high heat, about 5 minutes.

3. Pat dry the steaks and sprinkle them liberally with salt.

4. Once the pan is hot and just starting to smoke, drop in the fat and swirl to coat.

5. Place the steaks in the pan, presentation side down. Without touching them, sear for 3 to 4 minutes for a nice crust.

6. Flip over and sear for 3 to 4 minutes more, then set the steaks on a sheet pan.

7. Place the steaks in the oven. For medium-rare steaks, bake until the internal temperature is 125°F, about 8 minutes. For medium-done steaks, bake until the interior temperature is 135°F, about 10 minutes. Let the steaks rest for 5 to 10 minutes before serving.

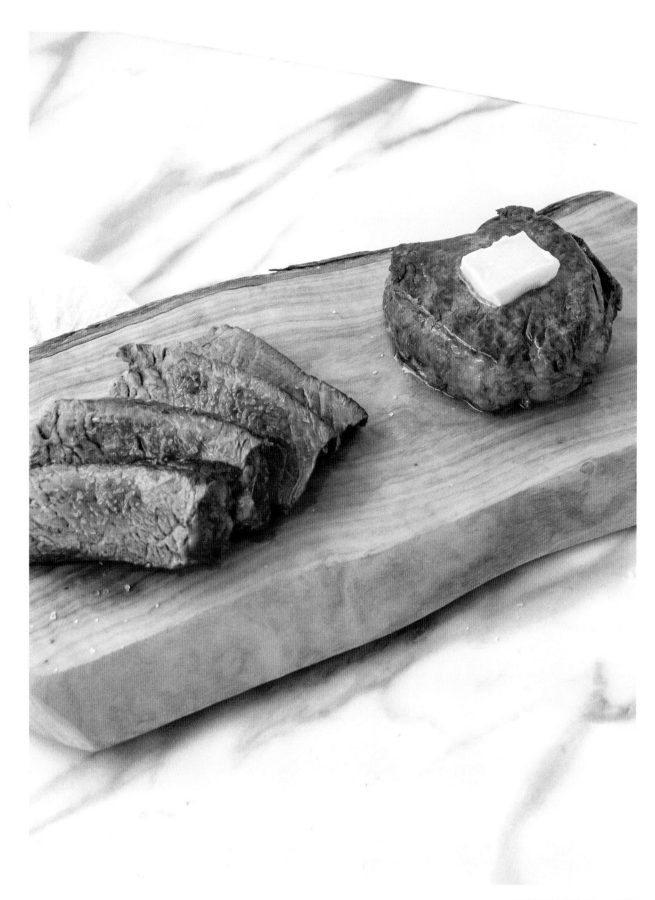

pot roast

YIELD:
4 to 6 servings

PREP TIME:
5 minutes

COOK TIME:
2 hours 40 minutes

This comforting dish is perfect for meal prep. While the recipe calls for a chuck roast, any tougher cut of beef, such as a rump or round roast, will work great for the braising method used here. Save tender cuts like beef tenderloin and rib eye steaks for quicker cooking methods such as pan-searing or grilling. Pan-searing this tougher cut before roasting gives it extra flavor. To make sure that flavor ends up in the meat and is not left in the pan, take care to scrape up all those delicious browned bits from the bottom when you deglaze the pan with liquid in Step 6. Slowly cooking the meat in a bit of liquid ensures that it stays moist and tender. When it's done, make sure to moisten the cooked meat with some of the flavorful cooking liquid, or make a yummy little sauce by whisking together some of the cooking liquid with sour cream until smooth.

1 (2½-pound) boneless chuck roast

2 teaspoons kosher salt

2 tablespoons tallow or other heat-tolerant fat of choice, for the pot

1 cup beef broth, homemade (page 126) or store-bought, or filtered water

1. Preheat the oven to 350°F.

2. Preheat a medium-size Dutch oven or other similarly sized lidded, oven-safe pot over medium-high heat.

3. Meanwhile, pat the meat dry and season it with the salt.

4. Once the pot is hot and just starting to smoke, drop in the tallow and swirl to coat.

5. Place the roast in the pot and sear until well browned on both sides, about 4 minutes per side.

6. Pour in the broth and scrape the bottom of the pot to release the browned bits, moving the chuck out of the way as needed.

7. Cover and place in the oven for about 2½ hours, flipping the meat over halfway through cooking, until cooked through and fork-tender. Serve a piece as is, or shred the meat.

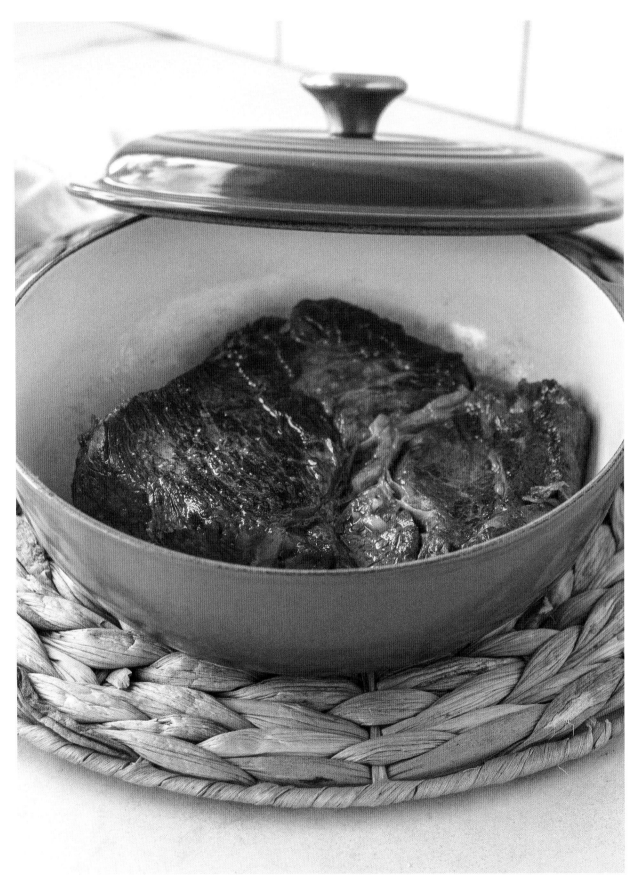

instant pot smoked brisket

YIELD:
6 to 8 servings

PREP TIME:
10 minutes

COOK TIME:
1 hour 20 minutes

Traditionally, smoked brisket is cooked low and slow all day in a smoker, but I'm just not that patient, especially when it comes to meat. This recipe uses an Instant Pot to speed up the cooking process. (If you are from Texas, please don't judge me.) The Instant Pot does double duty of searing the brisket and pressure-cooking it until tender. If your smoker has a grill, you could grill the meat instead of searing it in the Instant Pot.

I find that 30 minutes is enough time to give the meat that smoky flavor, but feel free to smoke it for a full hour if you like a lot of smoke. I will also add that using a smoker is not absolutely necessary. If you are not using a smoker, you can skip Steps 2 and 3, but I recommend using smoked salt to season the meat. That way, you'll still get a touch of smoke flavor. To make a simple sauce, use the cooking liquid as a broth and whisk in sour cream until thickened to your liking.

3 pounds brisket (see note)

Kosher salt

2 tablespoons tallow or other heat-tolerant fat of choice, for the pot

1. Cut the brisket into 3 to 4 strips or chunks. Liberally salt the meat on all sides.

2. Prep your smoker according to the manufacturer's instructions.

3. Smoke the brisket at 225°F for 30 minutes.

4. Turn an Instant Pot to the high heat sauté setting, drop in the tallow, and swirl to coat the pot.

5. Sear the brisket for 2 to 3 minutes on all sides, working in batches if needed to avoid crowding.

6. Once the searing is complete, add ½ cup of water to the pot, secure the lid, and set to pressure cook on high heat for 45 minutes.

7. When it is done cooking, allow the pressure to release naturally for 20 minutes.

8. Remove the brisket from the pot and carve off large pieces for serving, or shred it.

Note:

Most briskets come in 6- to 8-pound slabs. I break down the slab into roughly 3-pound portions and freeze them in zip-top bags for the next time I want to make brisket.

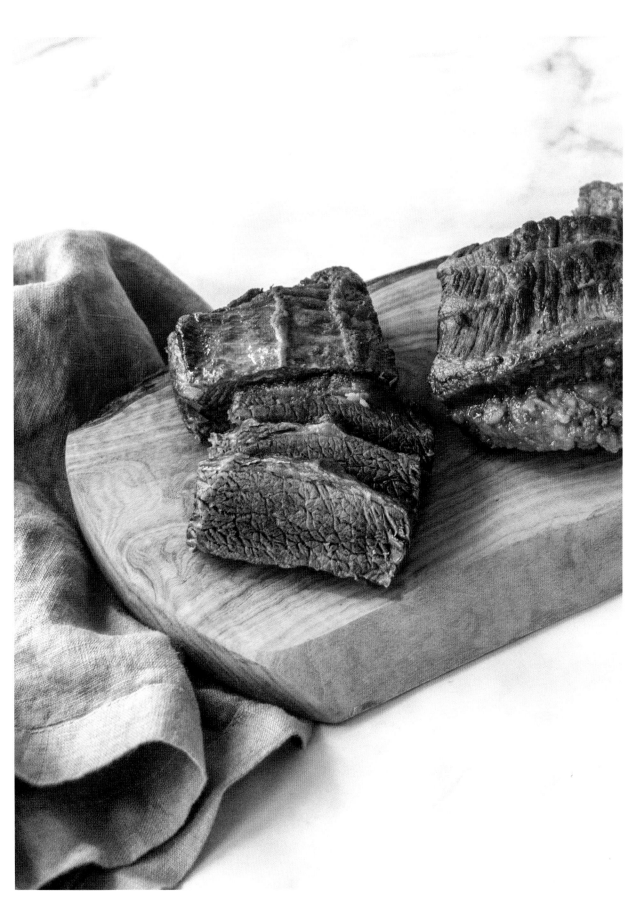

crispy chicken thighs

YIELD:
2 servings

PREP TIME:
5 minutes

COOK TIME:
25 minutes

I love how simple these little guys are. You can cook them in an air fryer if that is more up your alley (see the notes below). The average size of bone-in chicken thighs is about 6 ounces; if you use smaller thighs, remember that they may cook more quickly. Frying the chicken in bacon grease adds flavor, but you can use tallow if you avoid pork. Also, if you tolerate seasonings, I recommend using lemon pepper! These crispy thighs are tasty as is or served with a yummy sauce such as my Blue Cheese Cream Sauce (page 216) or Browned Butter Cream Sauce (page 206). If you pair them with a sauce and some noodles (see pages 92 to 95), you will likely be able to stretch the number of servings to three or four.

2 pounds bone-in, skin-on chicken thighs

Kosher salt

1 tablespoon bacon grease or other heat-tolerant fat of choice, for the pan

1. Preheat the oven to 400°F.

2. Preheat a large cast-iron skillet or other oven-safe skillet over medium-high heat until just beginning to smoke, about 5 minutes.

3. Pat dry the chicken and season both sides generously with salt.

4. Drop the bacon grease into the pan and swirl to coat the pan, then set the thighs in the pan, skin side down.

5. Cook for about 8 minutes, without touching, until there is a nice golden crust on the skin.

6. Flip the thighs over and immediately put the skillet in the oven.

7. Bake until cooked through, 18 to 20 minutes, depending on the size of the thighs. When done, the meat will no longer be pink at the center and the internal temperature will be 165°F. Serve immediately.

Notes:

To cook the thighs in an air fryer, preheat it to 400°F on the air fry setting. Drizzle some melted bacon grease on the chicken skin, then season the thighs with a generous sprinkling of salt. Bake them skin side up until cooked through, 20 to 25 minutes. When done, the meat will no longer be pink at the center and the internal temperature will be 165°F.

If doubling this recipe for the Dairy-Free Carnivore Meal Plan (see page 48), use two large skillets to avoid overcrowding, swapping the pans halfway through baking for even cooking.

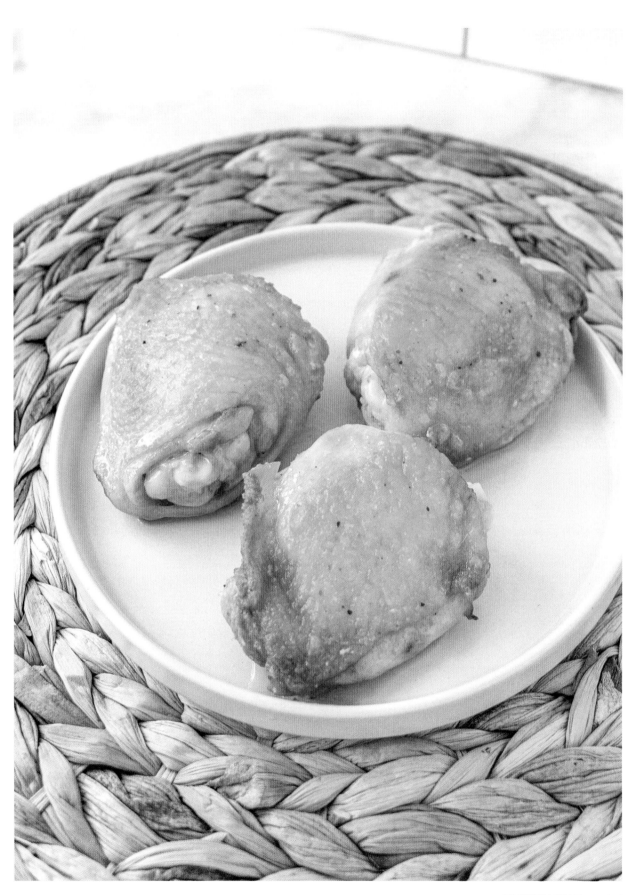

air fryer shrimp

YIELD:
2 servings

PREP TIME:
5 minutes

COOK TIME:
12 minutes

You can use any shrimp for this recipe, but I love using red Argentine shrimp. I call them lobster shrimp because they taste like lobster, but better. I also love how you can throw them into the air fryer straight from the freezer—super convenient! Eat them as is or serve with Panko Noodles (page 92) and Browned Butter Cream Sauce (page 206), as pictured.

1 pound frozen red Argentine shrimp or other jumbo shrimp, peeled and deveined

1 tablespoon salted butter, melted

Pinch of kosher salt

1. Preheat the air fryer to 400°F on the air fry setting.

2. Place the frozen shrimp on a baking tray and bake for 5 minutes. Drizzle on the butter, sprinkle lightly with salt, and stir well. Continue baking for another 5 to 7 minutes, until cooked through and opaque.

3. Serve immediately and enjoy!

Note:
I buy red Argentine shrimp at Costco, but they are available at other grocery stores and specialty seafood markets as well.

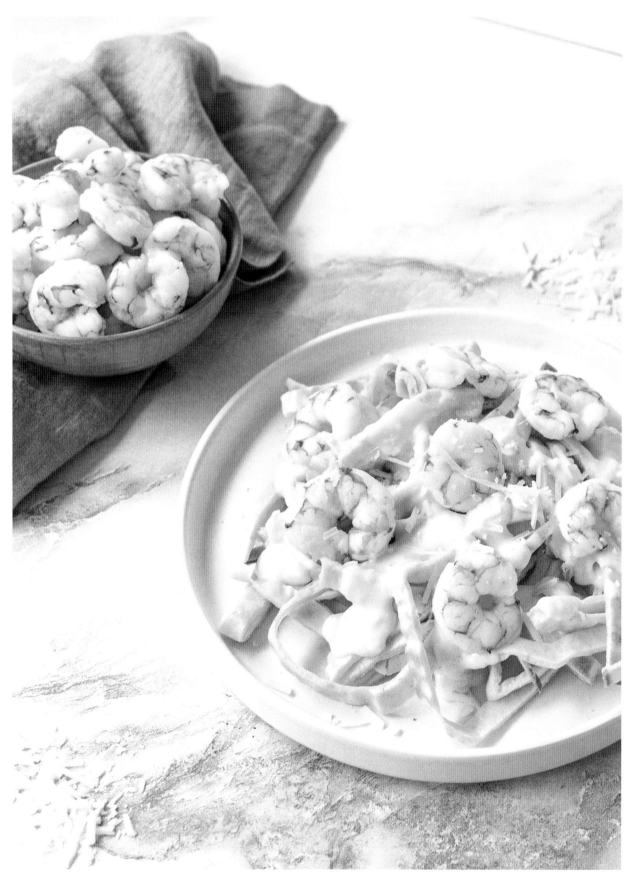

salmon bites

YIELD:
2 servings

PREP TIME:
10 minutes

COOK TIME:
6 minutes

When choosing salmon, wild caught is great, but I prefer farmed. There are some companies out there that practice sustainable farming (see "Shopping Tips" on page 24). I also like farmed salmon better because the fish tends to be fattier, which gives it a buttery-like finish. Leaner wild-caught salmon can be on the drier side. While I mainly stick to salt, a sprinkling of lemon pepper is a nice touch if you eat spices.

1 pound skinless salmon fillets, cut into 1-inch chunks

3 tablespoons salted butter, for the pan

Kosher salt

1. Preheat a large cast-iron skillet over medium-high heat for about 3 minutes.

2. When the pan is hot but not yet smoking, drop in the butter and swirl to coat the pan. Place the chunks of fish in the hot pan in a single layer. Sprinkle them lightly with salt.

3. Cook until a nice brown crust has formed, 2 to 3 minutes, then flip the pieces over and cook for another 2 to 3 minutes, until both sides are browned and the fish is just cooked through. You can check for doneness with a fork; if it's flaky, it's done.

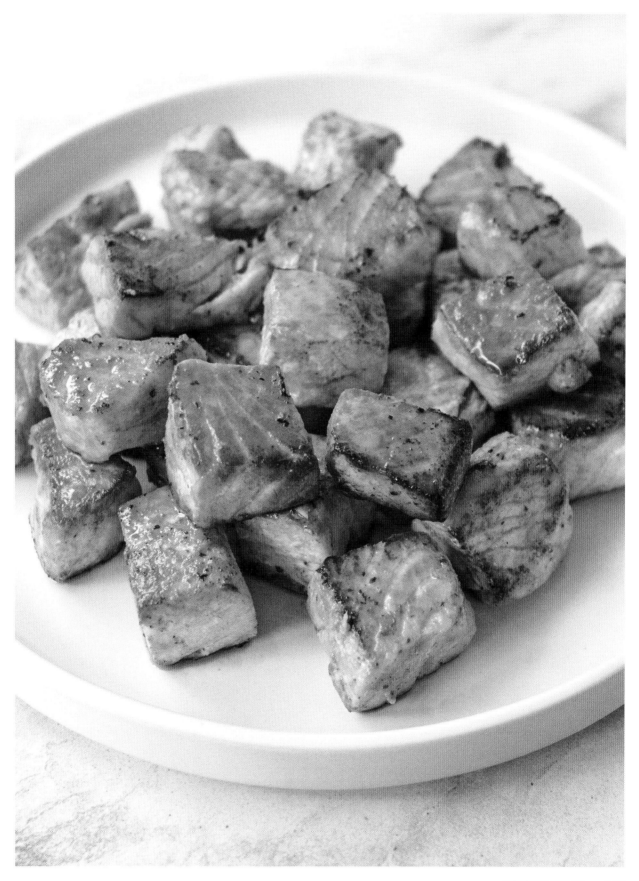

pan-seared chicken breast

YIELD:
2 servings

PREP TIME:
5 minutes

COOK TIME:
25 minutes

This easy and affordable dish is perfect for meal prep. I use a two-part cooking method here, searing the chicken on the stovetop first and then finishing it in the oven for even cooking and hands-off preparation time. I use this chicken for making Chicken Salad (page 130) or top it with a sauce, such as my Hollandaise (page 208) or Blue Cheese Cream Sauce (page 216). In my opinion, chicken breast needs a sauce. While it's fine to have leaner days occasionally, most people feel better when they eat more fat. Because chicken breast is extremely lean, it's wise to pair it with a fatty sauce.

1 pound boneless, skinless chicken breasts (see note)

Kosher salt

1 tablespoon tallow or other heat-tolerant fat of choice, for the pan

1. Preheat the oven to 400°F.

2. Preheat a large cast-iron skillet or other oven-safe pan over medium-high heat for about 5 minutes. While the pan heats, pat dry the breasts and season both sides liberally with the salt.

3. When the pan is hot and just starting to smoke, drop in the tallow and swirl to coat.

4. Place the chicken breasts in the pan, smooth presentation-side down. Sear until a nice golden crust forms, without touching the breasts, 6 to 8 minutes.

5. Once browned, flip the chicken breasts and immediately pop the pan into the oven.

6. Bake until cooked through, 18 to 20 minutes. When done, a thermometer will read 165°F when inserted in the thickest part of the breast.

7. Let rest on a cutting board for 5 minutes before slicing and serving.

Note:

The average size of boneless half-breasts (the single-serving portion) is between 6 and 8 ounces. If using smaller or larger breasts, adjust the cooking time accordingly.

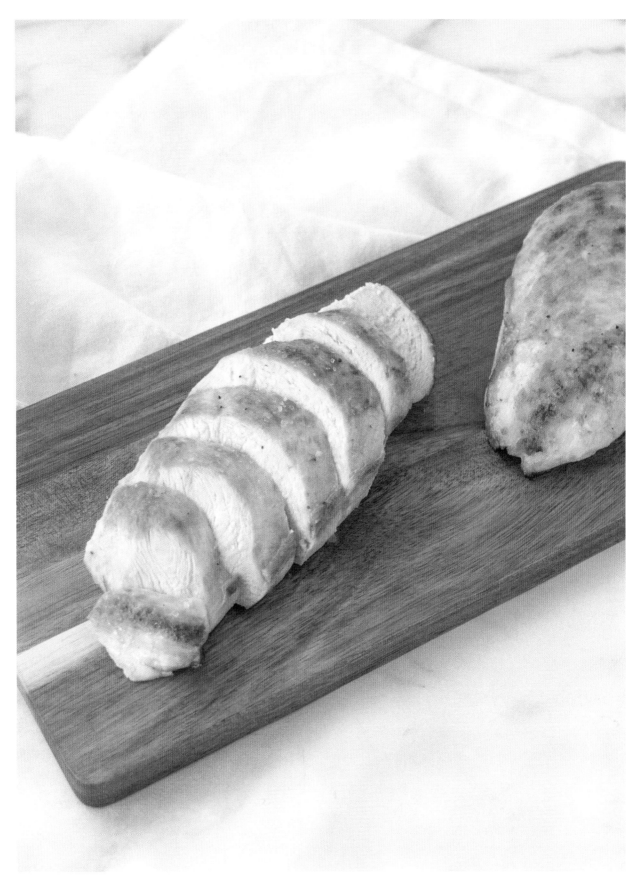

pan-seared scallops

YIELD:
2 servings as a main course or
4 servings as a starter

PREP TIME:
5 minutes

COOK TIME:
4 minutes

Scallops are one of my favorite types of seafood. I consider them the "butter of the sea" because they're so rich and tender. I recommend using this dish as an accompaniment to a steak for a wonderful surf-and-turf meal. You also could serve these scallops as a main course with Panko Noodles (page 92) and Browned Butter Cream Sauce (page 206) or place them on top of bacon pieces and serve them with a cream sauce as an appetizer.

1 pound sea scallops

Kosher salt

2 tablespoons salted butter, for the pan

1. Preheat a large cast-iron skillet over medium-high heat for about 3 minutes.

2. Pat dry the scallops and lightly sprinkle salt on both sides.

3. When the pan is hot but not yet smoking, drop in the butter and swirl to coat the pan.

4. Place the scallops in the pan, making sure to leave some space between them to avoid steaming. Depending on the size of your skillet, you may need to work in batches.

5. Sear undisturbed for 2 minutes on the first side to ensure a nice golden crust.

6. Flip and continue cooking for 1 to 2 minutes, until golden brown on both sides and opaque at the center.

7. Serve immediately.

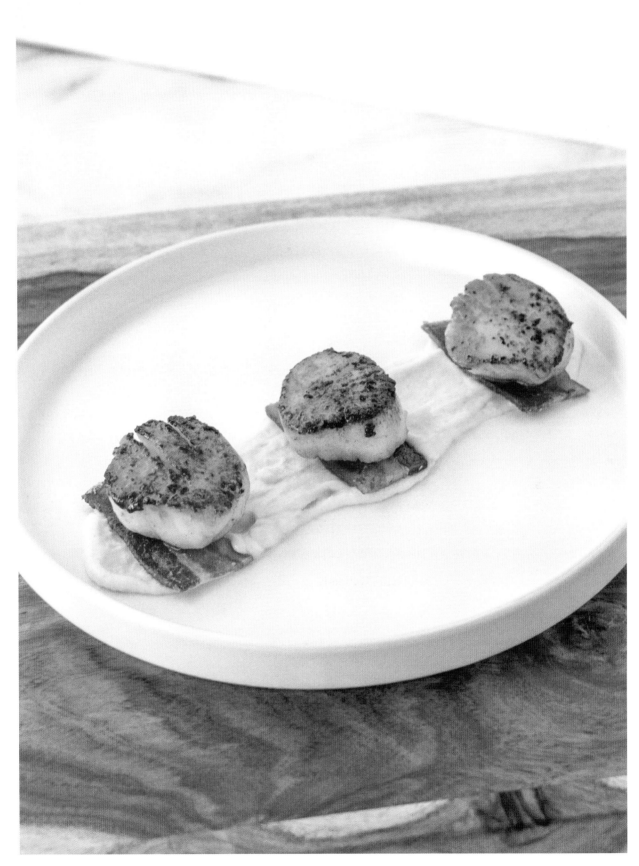

pan-seared rib eye

YIELD:
2 servings

PREP TIME:
5 minutes, plus 30 minutes to temper steak

COOK TIME:
10 minutes

The rib eye is arguably the best cut of steak because of its perfect ratio of fat to meat—not to mention the beauty that is the cap. In fact, during the holiday season, Costco sells just the caps! They are tender, fatty, and the most delicious bite of meat you could ever eat. Rib eyes are great as is, but to kick things up a notch, you can always top them with Blue Cheese Cream Sauce (page 216) or a simple pat of butter. I like to bring thick steaks to room temperature when they are not being finished in the oven to ensure that the center cooks properly without overcooking the exterior.

1 (1-pound) boneless rib eye, about 1½ inches thick (see notes)

Kosher salt

1 tablespoon salted butter, for the pan

1 tablespoon tallow or other heat-tolerant fat of choice, for the pan

1. Set the steak on the counter for about 30 minutes to bring it to room temperature.

2. Preheat a large cast-iron skillet over medium-high heat, about 5 minutes. While the pan is heating, pat the steak dry and salt it liberally.

3. Once the pan starts to smoke, drop in the butter and tallow and swirl to coat the pan.

4. Set the steak in the hot pan and allow to cook undisturbed for 3 minutes. Flip and cook for 3 more minutes without touching it.

5. Lower the heat to medium and cook, flipping the steak every minute, for an additional 4 minutes for medium-rare or up to 6 minutes for medium-done. For medium-rare, the internal temperature should be 125°F; for medium-done, 135°F. If you don't have a meat thermometer, you can use the finger touch to test doneness (see notes).

6. When the steak is done, remove it to a cutting board and let it rest for 5 to 10 minutes before cutting into it. (Being patient while it rests is the hardest part about cooking a steak!)

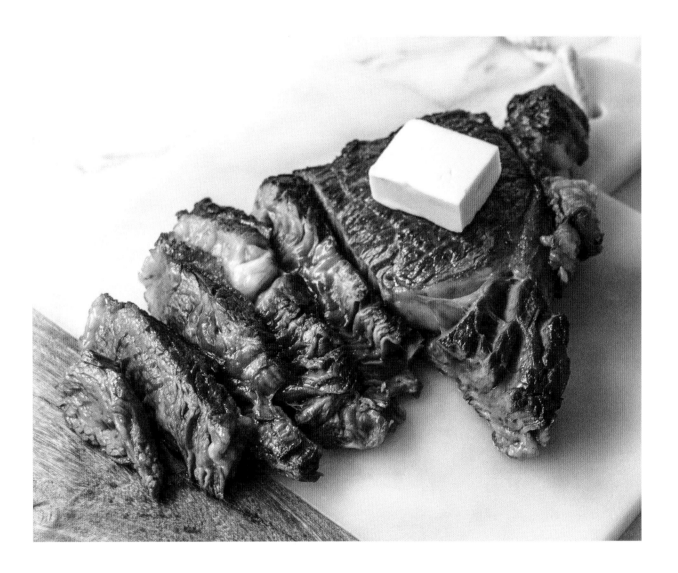

Notes:

If you have a thinner steak (¾ to 1 inch thick), the 6 minutes of cooking time over medium-high heat in Step 4 may be sufficient. To test doneness, follow the instructions in Step 5.

When dropped into a very hot skillet, butter will burn. The solution is to combine equal parts of butter and another, more heat-tolerant fat, like tallow.

A meat thermometer isn't required to test the doneness of steak—you can go a little rogue and use your finger. Lightly press your thumb and pointer finger together, then poke the pad of the palm under your thumb with your other hand. Note how soft/squishy it feels. Now touch the steak. Rare to medium-rare steak should have the same level of give. For medium-rare to medium steak, you can use the same technique, lightly pressing your thumb and middle finger to gauge the squishiness.

pan-seared skirt steak

YIELD:
4 servings

PREP TIME:
5 minutes

COOK TIME:
10 minutes

Skirt steak is one of the most underrated cuts—but don't let the secret out or stores will start raising the price. Skirt steak and flap meat (aka bottom sirloin butt) are very similar, so you can use them interchangeably here. They come in long, thin planks. While you can cook them like that, I like to cut them into smaller portions, which makes them a better fit for the skillet and helps them cook faster. These cuts are best enjoyed when cooked to medium-rare doneness so they don't become tough. I love topping the steak with Blue Cheese Cream Sauce (page 216).

2 pounds skirt steak or flap meat

Kosher salt

2 tablespoons tallow or other heat-tolerant fat of choice, for the pan

1. Preheat a large cast-iron skillet over medium-high heat until it just starts to smoke, about 5 minutes.

2. While the pan is heating, cut the steak into 4 equal portions. Pat the steaks dry and season moderately with salt.

3. Drop the tallow into the hot pan and swirl to coat, then add the steaks, working in batches so the pan is not crowded.

4. Cook undisturbed for 2 to 3 minutes so the first side can get a nice sear, then flip and cook for 2 to 3 more minutes for medium-rare doneness.

5. Before serving, slice the meat against the grain into strips.

Note:

While it's good practice to cut all steak against the grain, it's especially important with cuts like skirt steak and flap meat. They have more muscle fibers than other cuts of meat, so much so that you can easily see the grains running through the meat. Be sure to slice perpendicular to those fibers before plating the steak to ensure the steak will be tender.

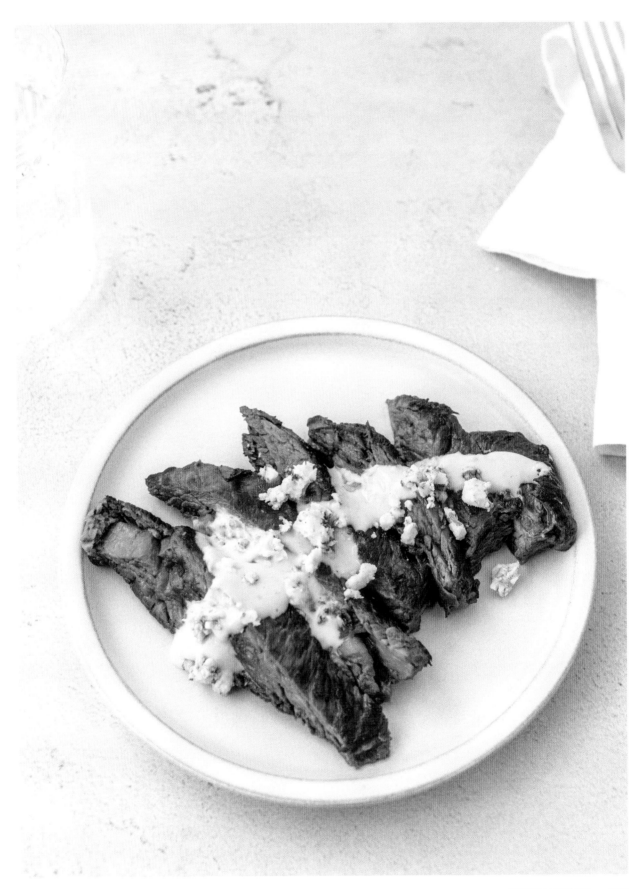

pan-seared heart

YIELD:
4 servings

PREP TIME:
5 minutes

COOK TIME:
8 minutes

If organs aren't your jam and you're eating them strictly for nutritional purposes, then you may want to think of this as a side dish rather than the main course. I suggest serving it alongside other meats, such as Crispy Chicken Thighs (page 140), Pan-Seared Skirt Steak (page 152), or Baked Bacon (page 166). I don't want to make you squirm, but you may see pieces that resemble tubes. Cut those off unless you're channeling your inner primal side. And just so I don't totally scare you away from trying this recipe, I'll add that because the heart is technically a muscle, you may find it to be more steak-like than liver, with a more palatable flavor than other organs. I recommend cooking heart to medium-rare to keep it tender; it can become tough and inedible if overcooked.

1 beef heart (about 2 pounds)

Kosher salt

1 tablespoon tallow or other heat-tolerant fat of choice, for the pan

1. Slice the heart into 4 steaks and trim off any tubes, exterior fat, or tough pieces.

2. Pat the steaks dry and lightly sprinkle salt on each side.

3. Preheat a large cast-iron skillet over medium-high heat for about 5 minutes. When smoking hot, drop in the tallow and swirl to coat the pan.

4. Place the steaks in the skillet, making sure not to crowd the pan to avoid steaming the steaks. Cook in batches, if needed. To ensure a nice sear, do not touch the steaks for a minimum of 2 minutes. Cook for 3 to 4 minutes on each side for medium-rare steaks.

You can ask your butcher or a local farmer to source beef heart for you, or you can find it at specialty meat purveyors, like Wild Fork (wildforkfoods.com), that carry a wide variety of meats, exotic cuts, and organs.

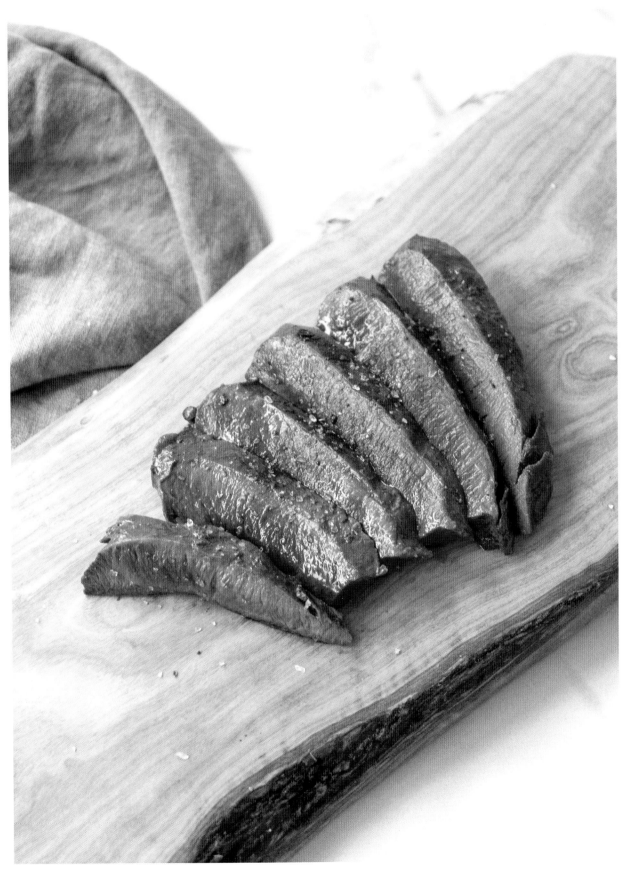

hidden liver burgers

YIELD:
4 patties (2 servings)

PREP TIME:
10 minutes

COOK TIME:
6 to 10 minutes, depending on desired doneness

We're not huge fans of liver at my house, but it's super nutritious, so I like to sneak some into our burgers. Even the kids love these! Be aware that adults shouldn't eat more than roughly 4 ounces of liver per week. It is very high in vitamin A, which can cause nausea and stomach issues, so you don't want to overdo it. I find it helpful to blend up the entire container of liver from the store, portion it into 4-ounce bags, and keep them in the freezer until I need them. You can serve these burgers as is or with your favorite burger toppings and All-Purpose Waffles (page 86) as buns. Note that if you serve them on waffle buns and bulk them out with bacon slices and/or cheese, you should be able to stretch the number of servings to four.

1 pound ground beef

4 ounces pureed beef liver (see notes)

1 large egg (see notes)

1 teaspoon kosher salt

1 teaspoon tallow or other heat-tolerant fat of choice, for the pan

1. Put the ground beef, pureed liver, egg, and salt in a medium-size bowl and mix with your hands until combined. Divide the mixture into 4 equal portions and shape them into patties, about 4 inches in diameter.

2. Preheat a large cast-iron skillet over medium-high heat until just beginning to smoke, about 5 minutes. Once hot, drop in the tallow and swirl to coat the pan.

3. Cook the patties for 3 to 4 minutes on each side, until a nice crust forms and the burgers are medium done; cook for about 5 minutes a side for well-done burgers. (Medium burgers will have a temperature of about 140°F; well-done burgers, about 160°F.) Serve immediately.

Notes:

To puree the livers, put them in a food processor or blender and pulse/puree for about 30 seconds, until smooth. Liver is very soft, so it breaks down easily.

To keep these burgers lion diet friendly, omit the egg.

Though I prefer my steaks cooked medium-rare, burgers are different. Because of the way the meat is processed—ground ahead of time—it can become contaminated with bacteria. So, for food safety reasons, it's best to cook burgers at least to medium. To be absolutely sure my burgers won't make me sick, I cook them until well-done.

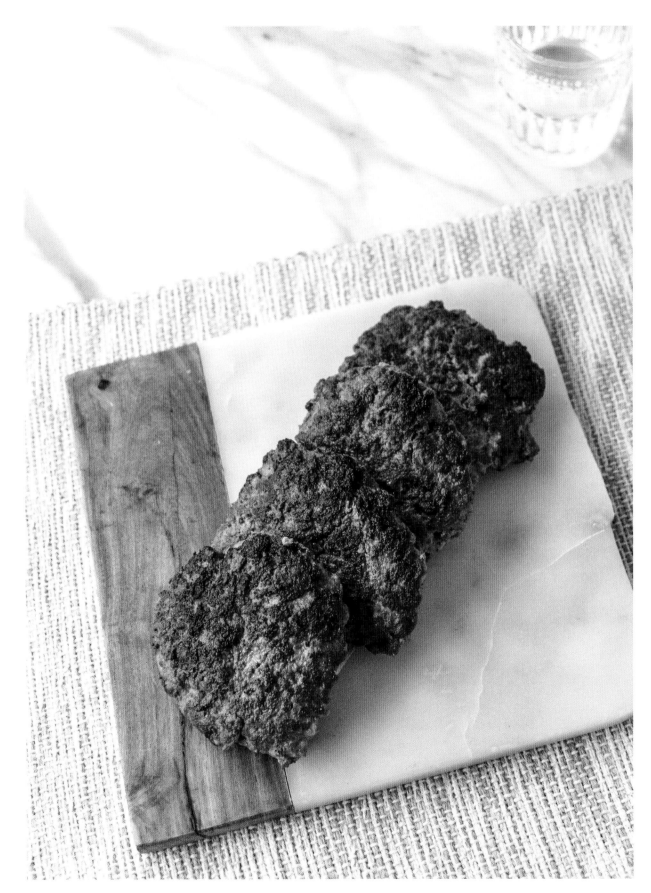

bacon-wrapped chicken thighs

YIELD:
3 servings

PREP TIME:
5 minutes

COOK TIME:
35 minutes

I love this fun way to jazz up chicken. Anything wrapped in bacon is delicious, right? Eat these thighs as is, or serve them with a sauce, such as Blue Cheese Cream Sauce (page 216). That combination will make you think of chicken wings with blue cheese dressing—only fancier.

6 boneless, skinless chicken thighs (about 1½ pounds)

Kosher salt

6 slices regular, thin-cut bacon

1. Preheat the oven to 400°F. Line a sheet pan with parchment paper.

2. Lightly salt the chicken. You will not want much because the bacon will be salty.

3. Take a slice of the bacon, stretch it to lengthen it a bit, and wrap it around a chicken thigh. Set the wrapped thigh on the prepared pan, making sure the ends are tucked under the bottom. Repeat with the remaining bacon slices and thighs.

4. Place the wrapped chicken pieces on the prepared pan.

5. Bake for 30 minutes or until the chicken reaches an internal temperature of 165°F.

6. Once cooked, remove from the oven and fry in a hot dry skillet over medium-high heat until the bacon is crisp, about 5 minutes. Alternatively, you can stick them under the broiler to brown.

Notes:

Regular, thin-cut bacon is ideal for this recipe; thick-cut bacon is too thick to wrap properly.

If choosing to fry the cooked thighs in a pan to crisp the bacon, you can begin heating the skillet about 5 minutes before the thighs come out of the oven. That way the skillet will be preheated and ready to use as soon as the thighs are done baking. A large cast-iron skillet is best here.

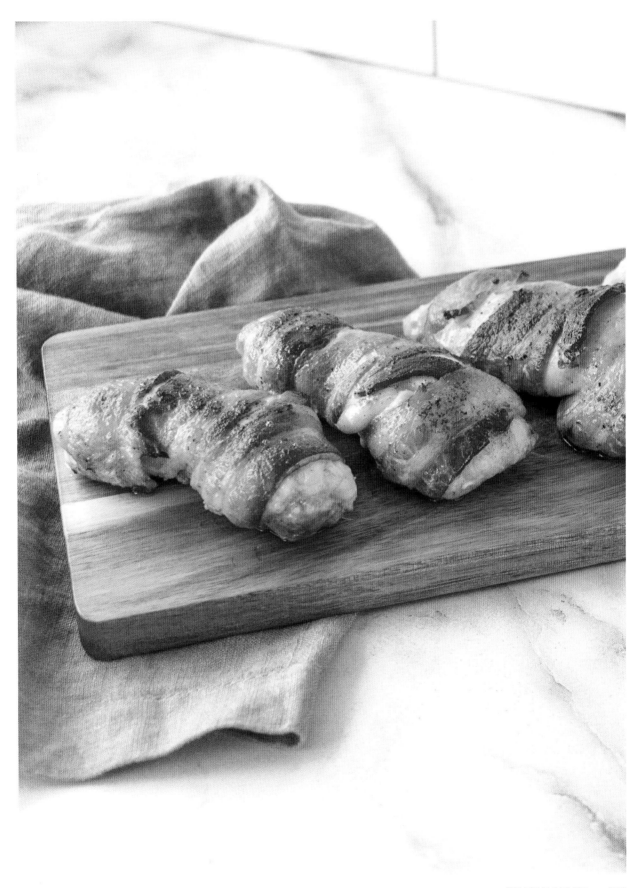

carnitas

YIELD:
8 servings

PREP TIME:
10 minutes

COOK TIME:
45 minutes or 5 to 10 hours, depending on method

Carnitas means little meats, and it is a traditional Mexican dish using a marbled cut of pork such as a boneless butt or shoulder. For this cut of pork, I recommend using the much faster Instant Pot method, but if you don't own one, you can also make this in a slow cooker. This recipe makes a large amount, which is great for serving guests or having easy meals for the week. We love using this meat for tacos, wrapped up in Tortillas (page 88) and topped with cheese and sour cream.

4 pounds boneless pork butt or shoulder, cut into 6 pieces, excess fat trimmed

2 teaspoons kosher salt

2 teaspoons ground cumin (optional)

1 cup chicken broth, homemade (page 126) or store-bought, or water

1. Put the meat in an Instant Pot or slow cooker. Sprinkle the meat with the salt and cumin, if using. Pour in the broth or water. If using a slow cooker, skip ahead to Step 3.

2. If using the Instant Pot, secure the lid and select pressure cook on high heat for 45 minutes. Allow the pressure to release naturally for 20 minutes. After the natural release is completed, carefully flip the valve and release the rest of the pressure.

3. If using a slow cooker, cover and cook on low for 8 to 10 hours or on high 5 to 7 hours. When done, the meat will be fork-tender.

4. Shred the meat with 2 forks in the cooking liquid.

5. Remove the shredded meat with a slotted spoon and place onto a sheet pan. Spread the meat into an even layer.

6. Place an oven rack in the top position and set the oven to the broiler setting. Broil the pork for about 15 minutes, stirring every 5 minutes. You want the ends of the meat pieces to get crispy while the rest of the meat stays moist. You can also use the broil setting in an air fryer to crisp the meat; however, given the smaller size of an air fryer, you'll need to work in batches to avoid overcrowding the meat.

7. Serve as is or make tacos!

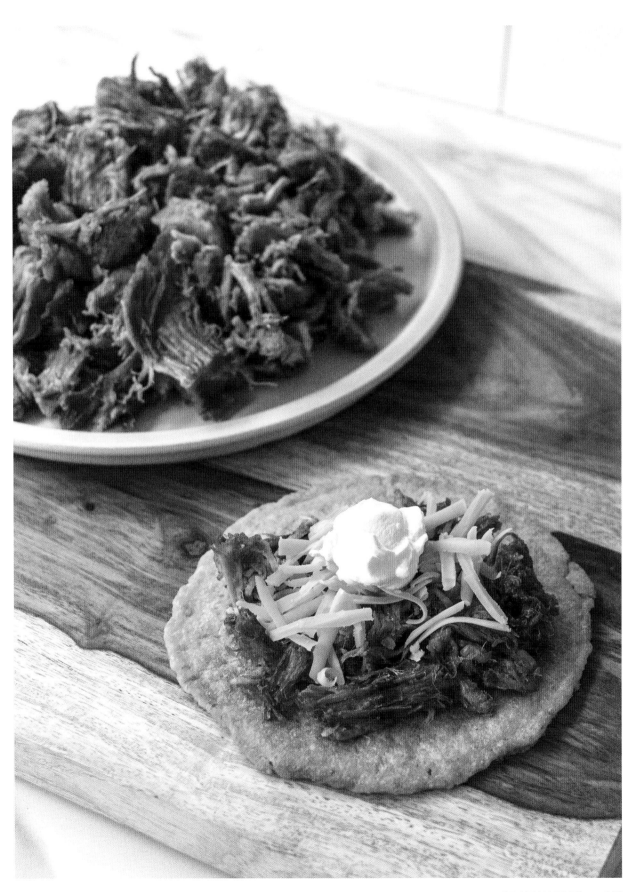

kofta meatballs

YIELD:
16 (2-inch) meatballs
(4 servings as a main course or
8 servings as a starter)

PREP TIME:
10 minutes

COOK TIME:
13 to 20 minutes, depending on
method

Kofta kebabs are a popular dish in the Middle East and Mediterranean. Being a Greek girl myself, I've always loved warmly spiced meats and, of course, feta cheese. Here, I've changed up the classic meat-on-a-stick by making cute little meatballs. I recommend serving these with my Creamy Feta Dip. However, they're very good on their own, too, so if you're looking for a meat-only meal without any added animal products, you may prefer to enjoy the meatballs as is. If you are strict carnivore and are not using seasonings, the meatballs are still delicious without the cinnamon and cumin. If you tolerate some plant foods and want to give the dish a bit of warmth, though, I recommend including the spices. The meat mixture also makes great burger patties.

1 pound ground beef

1 pound ground lamb

2 teaspoons kosher salt

1 teaspoon ground
cinnamon (optional)

½ teaspoon ground cumin
(optional)

Creamy Feta Dip (page
212), for serving (optional)

1. Preheat the oven or an air fryer on the air fry setting to 425°F.

2. Put the beef, lamb, salt, and spices (if using) in a large bowl and mix together with your hands.

3. Divide the meat mixture in half, then in half again, to make 4 equal portions. Roll 4 equal-sized meatballs from each portion, for a total of 16 meatballs.

4. If using the air fryer, place the meatballs in the basket and air-fry for 13 to 15 minutes, or until cooked through. If using the oven, place the meatballs on a sheet pan and bake for 18 to 20 minutes, or until cooked through. When cooked through, they will no longer be pink in the center, and the internal temperature will be 160°F.

5. Serve immediately, along with the dip, if using.

Note:

To experiment with the seasonings, after completing Step 2, fry up one little piece of the seasoned meat mixture in a skillet. Taste-test the cooked meat, and then add more salt, cinnamon, and/or cumin to the mixture if needed before shaping the meatballs.

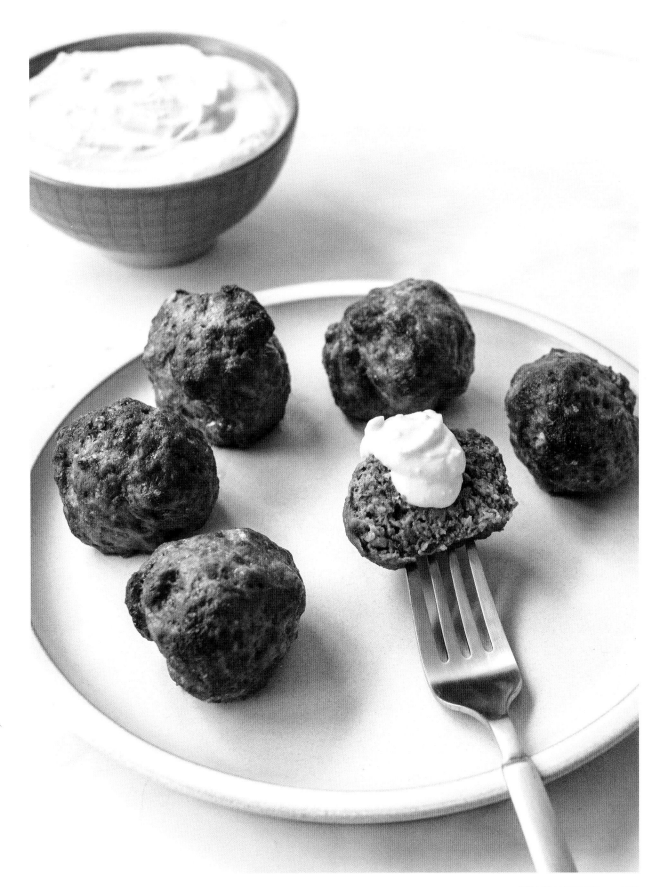

lamb lollipops

YIELD:
2 servings as a main course or
4 to 6 servings as a starter

PREP TIME:
5 minutes

COOK TIME:
10 minutes

Eating meat right off the bone just feels so primal. These lamb lollipops are fun to eat and are best paired with my Creamy Feta Dip (page 212). Serve them as an entrée or as an appetizer—they make a perfect finger food when you're entertaining guests. Racks of lamb vary in size from 1 to 2 pounds; depending on what's available at your market, you can easily scale this recipe up or down as needed.

1 frenched rack of lamb
(about 1½ pounds)

Kosher salt

1 tablespoon tallow or
other heat-tolerant fat of
choice, for the pan

1. Slice between each rib bone of the rack of lamb, cutting all the way through to make a small lamb chop, or lollipop.

2. Pat dry and salt each side.

3. Preheat a large cast-iron skillet over medium-high heat until it starts to smoke, about 5 minutes.

4. Drop in the tallow and swirl to coat the pan. Place half of the lollipops in the pan and cook for 2 to 3 minutes on each side for medium-rare/ medium-done chops. Do not touch the chops for at least 2 minutes to ensure a good sear.

5. Cook the remainder of the lollipops and serve immediately.

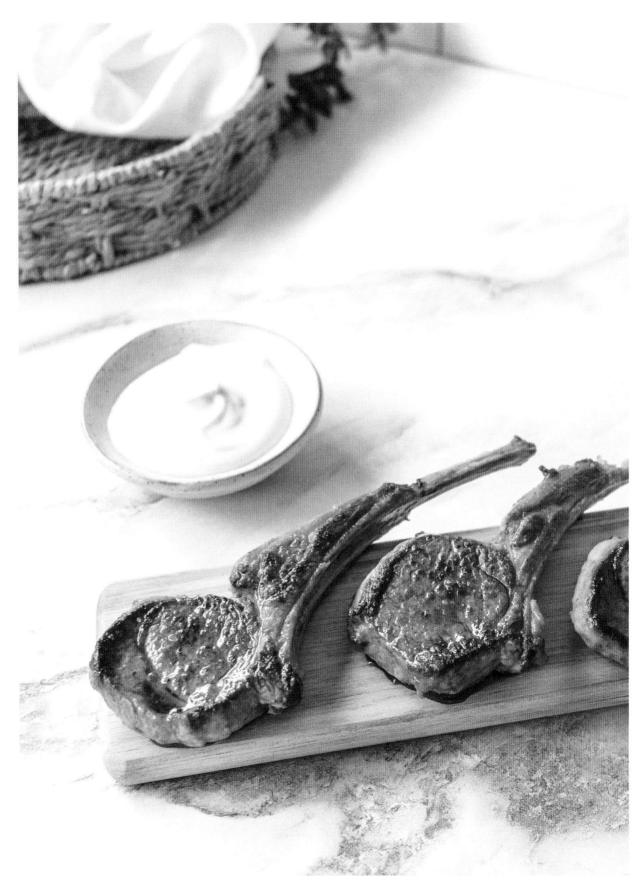

baked bacon

YIELD:
4 servings

PREP TIME:
5 minutes

COOK TIME:
25 minutes

This is the easiest, cleanest way to make bacon! No more babysitting it on the stove, flipping it, and getting popped in the face with grease. With this oven method, the bacon cooks nice and flat, and the fat will melt in your mouth. Save the grease in a ramekin and use it to cook other things or to make Butter Bacon Mayonnaise (page 210). Half a pound of bacon will give you approximately ¼ cup of grease.

This method can be used for either thin- or thick-cut bacon. I use thin-cut bacon and, for portioning purposes, specify that cut of bacon in most of the recipes. Unless a recipe requires thin-cut bacon, feel free to use thick-cut if that is your preference; in that case, you can use fewer slices than what's called for in the recipes since thick-cut bacon is so much heartier. Note that if you're a fan of crispy bacon, thin-cut is for you; if you like chewy bacon, go with thick-cut (again, unless the recipe requires thin-cut).

8 ounces bacon (any thickness)

1. Turn the oven on to 400°F. Line a sheet pan with parchment paper.

2. Lay the slices of bacon out on the prepared pan and put in the oven; no need to wait for the oven to come to temperature.

3. Cook for 20 to 25 minutes, depending on the thickness of bacon you're using and the doneness you like.

4. Save the grease to use later!

Note:

If you cook a full pound of bacon, you will need two sheet pans. Switch the pans on the racks halfway through. You might also need to bump up the cooking time a bit, closer to 30 minutes.

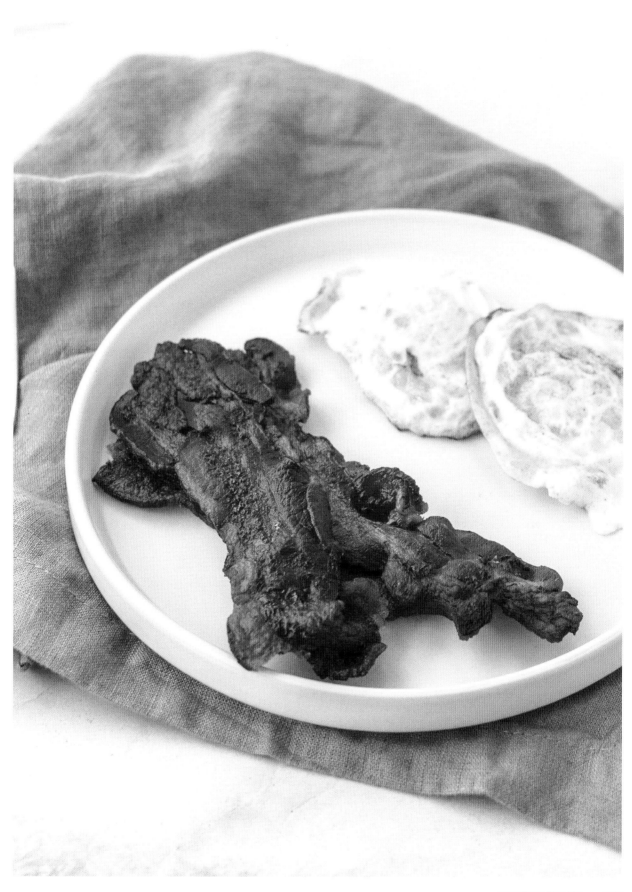

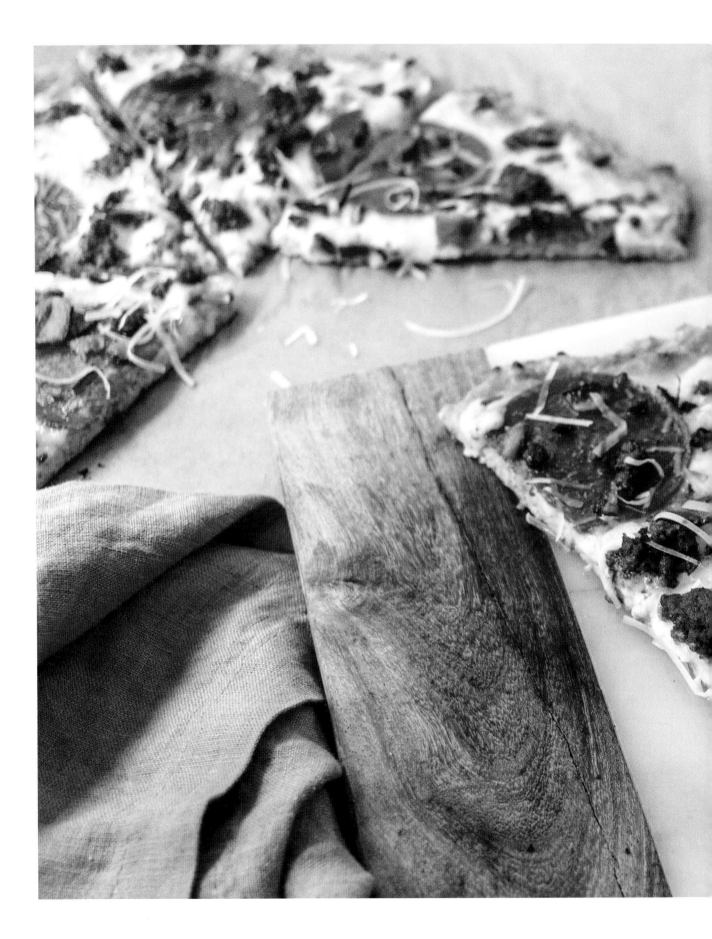

comforting classics

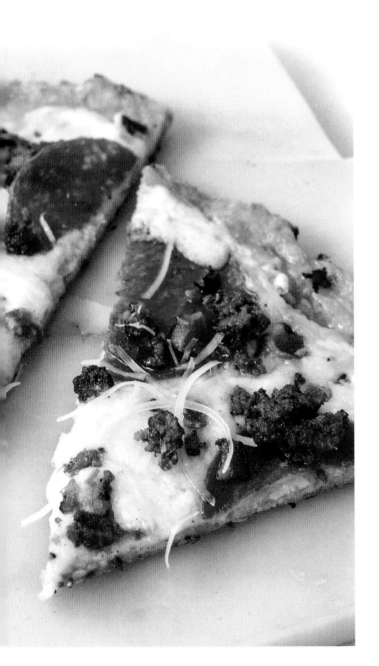

creamy chicken casserole *with* crunchy panko topping

YIELD:
6 servings

PREP TIME:
10 minutes (not including time to cook chicken)

COOK TIME:
30 minutes

Back in the day, I used to make a comfort food dish called Poppyseed Chicken. It was a creamy, gooey, chicken-y casserole topped with crushed buttery crackers and sprinkled with—you guessed it—poppyseeds. These days, I swap the crackers for pork panko and leave the seeds for the birds. I hope this dish feels like a warm hug (unless you're not a hugger).

1 (8-ounce) package cream cheese, softened

1 cup sour cream

½ cup heavy cream

4 cups finely chopped cooked chicken breast (see notes)

FOR THE TOPPING:

¾ cup pork panko

2 tablespoons salted butter, melted

½ cup pregrated Parmesan cheese (see notes)

1. Preheat the oven to 375°F.

2. Put the cream cheese, sour cream, and heavy cream in a large bowl. Mix well, then stir in the chicken. Transfer the mixture to an 11 by 7-inch casserole dish.

3. To make the topping, put the panko and melted butter in a small bowl and mix well. Add the Parmesan and stir to combine. Sprinkle the mixture on top of the chicken mixture.

4. Bake for 25 to 30 minutes, until hot and bubbly.

Notes:

To get the 4 cups of finely chopped cooked chicken needed for this recipe, cook about 2 pounds of raw boneless, skinless chicken breasts. You can use any cooking method you like; to pan-sear it, see the recipe on page 146.

To ensure that the casserole topping stays nice and crunchy, I use pregrated shelf-stable Parmesan sold in jars or cans; shredded bagged Parmesan, sold in the refrigerated section of the grocery store, has too much moisture for this purpose. Shredded Parmesan will give you a melty cheese topping instead of a crunchy one.

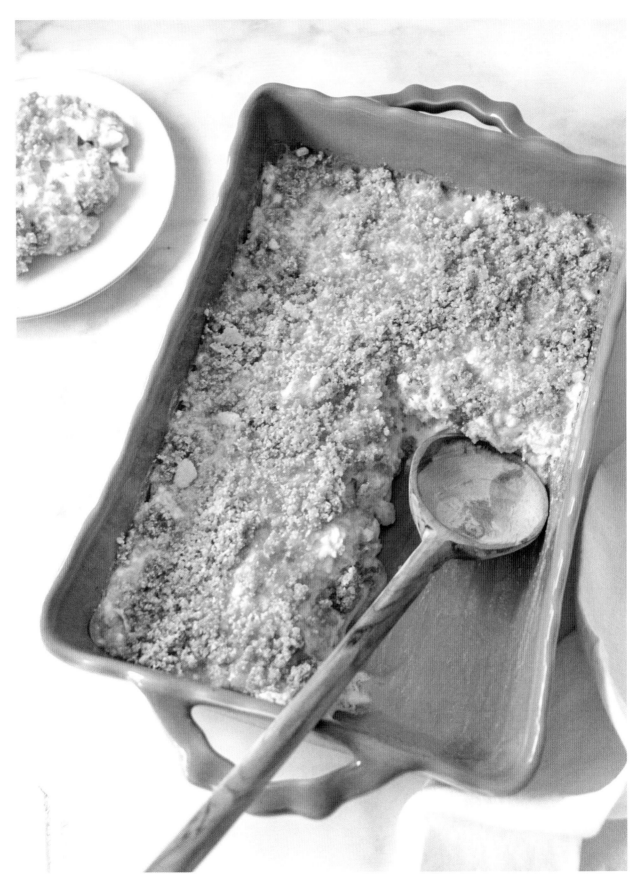

meatloaf

YIELD:
4 servings

PREP TIME:
10 minutes

COOK TIME:
75 minutes

Is it still meatloaf if it doesn't have a sugary ketchup glaze on top? I think so, and it's better for you, too. But if you top it with some ketchup, I won't judge. The Italian seasoning is optional if you can't tolerate it. If you can, it makes for a nice change from plain burger meat.

2 pounds ground beef

2 large eggs

⅓ cup heavy cream

¾ cup pork panko

1 teaspoon Italian seasoning (optional)

½ teaspoon kosher salt

1. Preheat the oven to 350°F.

2. Put the beef, eggs, and cream in a large bowl and mix with your hands until well combined.

3. In a small bowl, whisk together the pork panko, Italian seasoning (if using), and salt.

4. Add the dry ingredients to the wet and mix with your hands until evenly combined.

5. Put the meat mixture in a 9 by 5-inch loaf pan and smooth the top.

6. Bake for 75 minutes, or until the meat is cooked through. To test for doneness, insert a meat thermometer in the center of the loaf; it should read 160°F.

7. Let the meatloaf rest for 10 minutes before slicing and serving.

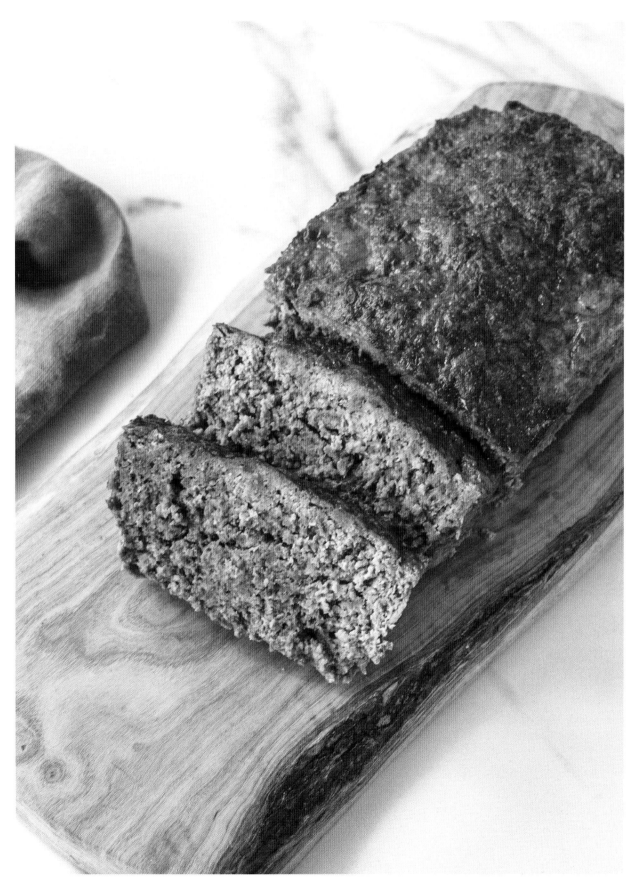

chili

YIELD:
6 servings

PREP TIME:
10 minutes

COOK TIME:
55 minutes

Who doesn't love a hearty bowl of chili in the wintertime? I love serving this chili with Cornbread Muffins (page 90). It's a stick-to-your-ribs kind of meal that leaves you feeling nourished and satisfied. This chili also reheats wonderfully and makes for a great meal prep option. I recommend cooking the bacon in the oven; because it's a hands-off method, it allows you to proceed with the rest of the recipe and save time. However, if you'd like to cook the bacon on the stovetop, I've included instructions, opposite. Cooking the bacon that way will add 30 minutes to the total cook time for this recipe.

1 pound bacon

1 tablespoon tallow or bacon grease, for the pot

1 pound boneless sirloin, cut into bite-size chunks

1 pound ground beef

1 teaspoon ground cumin (optional)

1 teaspoon chili powder (optional)

2 cups beef broth, homemade (page 126) or store-bought

Kosher salt

SUGGESTED TOPPINGS:

Shredded semi-firm cheese, such as cheddar

Sour cream

Cooked bacon pieces (reserved from above)

1. Cook the bacon in the oven, following the directions in the Baked Bacon recipe (see page 166). Or cook the bacon on the stovetop (see the note, opposite).

2. While the bacon is cooking, preheat a medium-size Dutch oven or similarly sized soup pot over medium-high heat until hot and just beginning to smoke.

3. Once hot, drop in the fat and swirl to coat the pot. Add the sirloin and brown for 2 to 3 minutes to get a nice sear, then flip the chunks and sear the other side, another 2 to 3 minutes. Remove the sirloin and set aside.

4. To the pot, add the ground beef and spices (if using) and cook while breaking the meat apart until it is cooked through and browned, about 15 minutes.

5. Return the sirloin to the pot and add the broth.

6. Bring to a boil, then lower the heat and simmer, uncovered, until the sirloin is tender and the flavors have married, about 30 minutes.

7. When the bacon is done, break it into small pieces and add them to the simmering pot, saving about ¼ cup for topping, if desired.

8. Before serving, add salt to taste. The bacon adds a lot of salt, and depending on how your broth is salted, you may not need much additional salt, if any. Keep in mind the extra salt that will be added if topping with reserved bacon.

9. Serve garnished with your favorite toppings! We love using cheddar cheese, sour cream, and crumbled bacon.

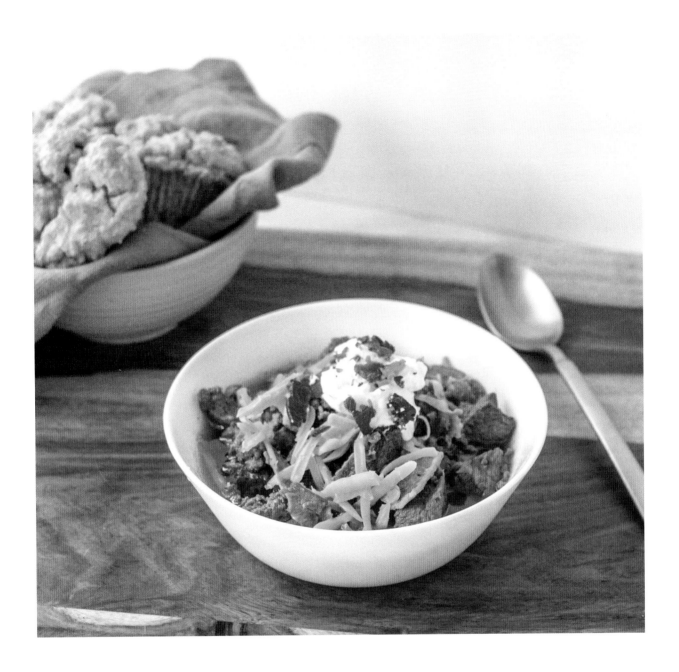

Note: To cook the bacon on the stovetop, cut it into small pieces (about 1 inch) and cook in a medium-size Dutch oven or similarly sized soup pot over medium heat, stirring occasionally, until crispy, about 30 minutes. Remove the bacon from the pot with a slotted spoon, then pour off all but about 1 tablespoon of the grease from the pot. If desired, set aside ¼ cup of the bacon pieces for topping the finished chili. Turn the heat up to medium-high and add the sirloin to the pot, searing it per the instructions in Step 3. Finish the recipe as written, adding the cooked bacon pieces to the pot after completing Step 6, when the meat is tender.

white lasagna

YIELD:
8 servings

PREP TIME:
15 minutes (not including time to make noodles and sauce)

COOK TIME:
55 minutes

Lasagna is one of my favorite comfort foods, so this dish just feels comfy-cozy to the soul. My whole family loves it, and it leaves us with plenty of leftovers. Of course, it's a little different from regular lasagna. Instead of using tomato sauce, I use my Browned Butter Cream Sauce, which is so delightful. If you're avoiding herbs and spices, omit the sausage and double the quantity of ground beef.

Double batch Panko Noodles (page 92), kept in sheet form

1 pound bulk Italian sausage

1 pound ground beef

1 batch Browned Butter Cream Sauce (page 206)

Kosher salt

3 cups shredded mozzarella cheese (about 12 ounces), divided

1 (15-ounce) container ricotta cheese

2 large eggs, whisked

½ cup shredded Parmesan cheese (about 1½ ounces)

1. Preheat the oven to 400°F. Trim the sheets of noodles to fit a 13 by 9-inch casserole dish; set the noodles and dish aside.

2. In a large skillet over medium-high heat, cook the meat, stirring to break it apart, until browned and cooked through, about 15 minutes. Drain the grease and add the sauce. Add salt to taste, if needed.

3. In a medium-size bowl, combine 1½ cups of the mozzarella, the ricotta, eggs, and Parmesan, making sure the cheeses and eggs are well blended.

4. In the casserole dish, layer half of the meat sauce, one sheet of noodle, and then half of the cheese mixture. Repeat with the remaining meat sauce, sheet of noodle, and cheese mixture. Top with the remaining 1½ cups of mozzarella.

5. Bake uncovered for 35 to 40 minutes, until the top is browned.

6. Let the lasagna rest for 5 minutes before cutting and serving.

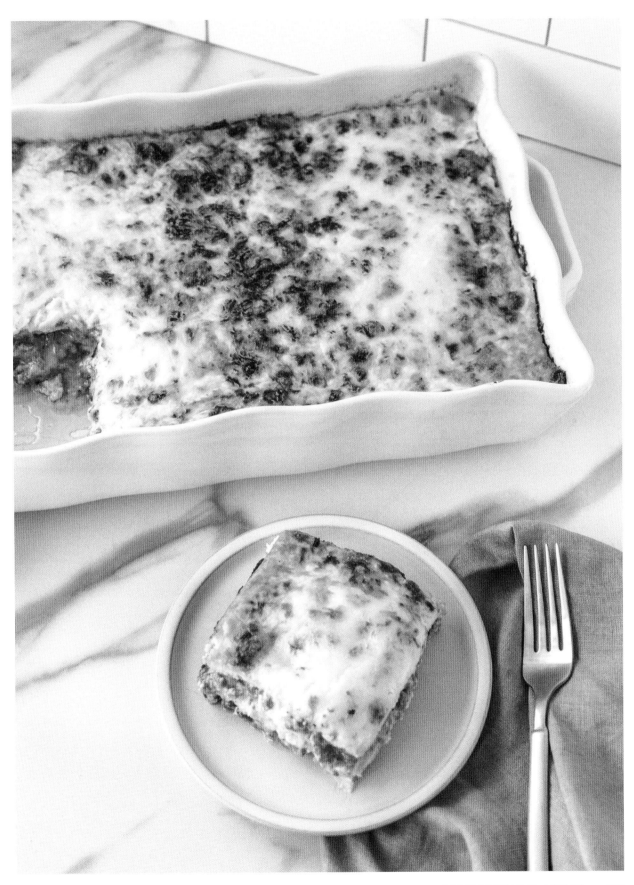

country-fried steak *with* gravy

YIELD:
2 servings

PREP TIME:
10 minutes

COOK TIME:
15 minutes

Country-fried steak is traditionally made with cubed steak, which is top round or top sirloin that has been run through a tenderizer. It tends to be a budget-friendly cut. It's typically very thin—¼ inch—and meant to be cooked quickly so it doesn't become tough. This is my twist on the old favorite. You can easily stretch this dish to serve four people by adding a side of fried eggs (see page 60) to each plate.

⅓ cup tallow or other heat-tolerant fat of choice, plus extra if needed, for the pan

4 cubed steaks (about 1 pound)

Kosher salt

1 large egg

1¼ cups pork panko

1 cup heavy cream

1. Heat the tallow in a large cast-iron skillet over medium-high heat, about 5 minutes. To test the heat level of the fat, drop a pinch of panko into the pan; if the panko sizzles, the fat is ready. Meanwhile, bread the steaks. (*Note:* If the fat comes to temperature before all the steaks are breaded, temporarily lower the heat.)

2. Pat dry the steaks and lightly sprinkle with salt.

3. Crack the egg into a medium-size bowl and whisk well.

4. Put the pork panko in a medium-size dish.

5. Take a steak and dip it in the egg to coat, letting the excess drip off. Press the steak into the panko and flip to coat both sides. Let any excess fall back into the bowl. Place the breaded steak on a plate and repeat with the remaining steaks.

6. Fry the breaded steaks for 2 to 3 minutes on each side, until golden brown. If your pan isn't large enough to cook them all without crowding, cook them in batches, checking the fat level as you work. Make sure the fat comes almost halfway up the sides of the steaks. If you add more fat, allow it to come to temperature before frying the next batch of steaks.

7. Place the cooked steaks on a wire rack and tent them with foil to keep warm while you make the gravy.

8. Slowly pour all but 1 tablespoon of fat from the pan, leaving all the browned bits at the bottom of the pan. Add the cream and whisk, scraping the bottom of the pan to release the browned bits.

9. Cook over medium-high heat, letting the gravy boil lightly and whisking frequently, until thickened, 6 to 7 minutes. Add salt to taste.

10. Plate the steaks and pour the gravy over them.

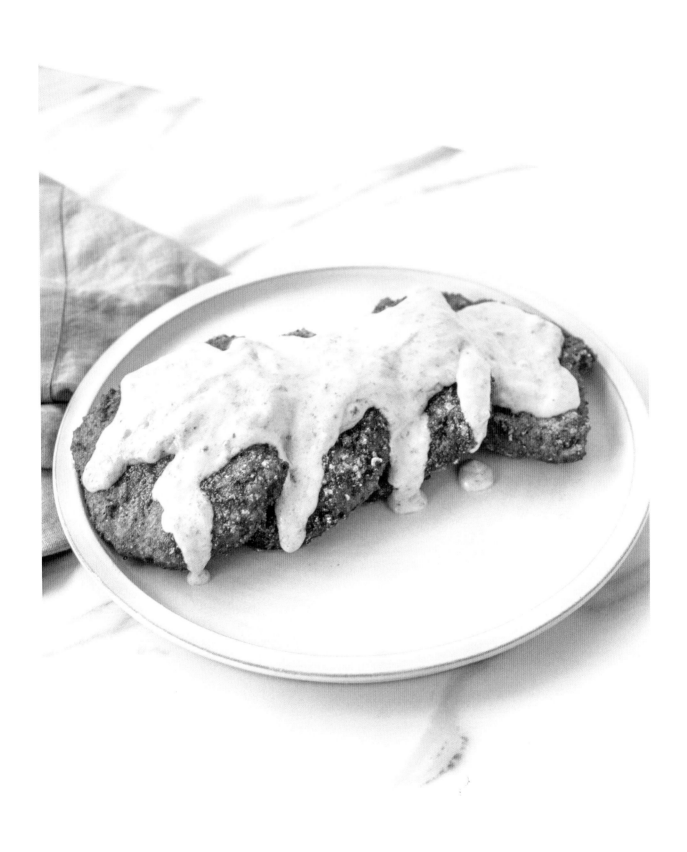

swedish meatballs

YIELD:
16 (1½-inch) meatballs
(2 servings)

PREP TIME:
10 minutes

COOK TIME:
30 minutes

Have you ever driven to IKEA just for the meatballs? Yeah, me too. Then I discovered I could save time by making them at home. These meatballs taste way better, they're better for you, and you won't end up with a piece of furniture with 837 components to assemble! Of course, Dijon mustard and pumpkin pie spice don't come from an animal, but if you tolerate spices, I highly suggest including them for a nice flavor change. If you're in a rush, you don't even have to form the mixture into balls. Simply omit the egg, pan-fry the seasoned meat, and serve it with the gravy poured over it. It's just as delicious! I typically eat this dish as is, but it is also great spooned over Panko Noodles (page 92) or Egg White Noodles (page 94), which would enable you to stretch this recipe to serve four people.

FOR THE GRAVY:

2 cups chicken broth, homemade (page 126) or store-bought

½ cup sour cream

¼ cup heavy cream

1 teaspoon Dijon mustard

Kosher salt

FOR THE MEATBALLS:

1 pound ground beef

1 large egg

1 teaspoon kosher salt

¼ teaspoon pumpkin pie spice

1 tablespoon tallow or other heat-tolerant fat of choice, for the pan

1. In a small saucepan, combine all the gravy ingredients, except the salt.

2. Bring to a boil over medium-high heat, stirring occasionally. Let it boil gently until the gravy is slightly reduced and thickened, 20 to 25 minutes. When done, add salt to taste, if needed.

3. While the gravy is doing its thing, start the meatballs. Put the beef, egg, salt, and pumpkin pie spice in a large bowl and mix well with your hands.

4. Separate the meat mixture into 4 equal portions, then take each portion and divide it in fourths, for a total of 16 pieces. Form those pieces into balls.

5. Heat a large cast-iron skillet over medium-high heat until just beginning to smoke. Drop in the tallow and swirl to coat the pan.

6. Cook the meatballs for a total of 8 minutes, or until nicely browned, turning them about every 2 minutes to hit all the sides.

7. Turn the heat down to medium and let the meatballs cook through, turning occasionally, 4 to 6 minutes more. When cooked through, they will no longer be pink in the center, and the internal temperature will be 160°F.

8. Serve immediately with the gravy poured over the meatballs.

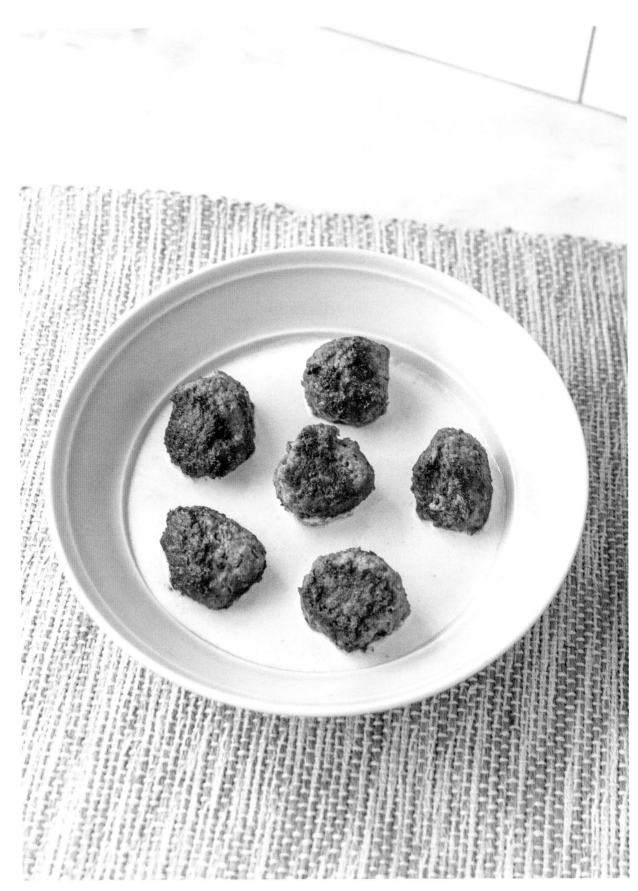

carnizza

YIELD:
1 (12-inch) pizza
(2 to 4 servings)

PREP TIME:
10 minutes

COOK TIME:
20 minutes

I let my Instagram community name this recipe, so if you think it's a corny title, blame them! You might be surprised by how much this tastes like regular pizza. If you've dabbled in keto cooking at all, you may have heard of fathead dough. In this take, I swap out the almond flour for pork panko. You can top the crust with my Browned Butter Cream Sauce (page 206) or live on the edge and use a tomato-based pizza sauce; I use sugar-free ketchup when serving it to my kids. Very gourmet, I know.

FOR THE CRUST:

1½ cups shredded mozzarella cheese (about 6 ounces)

1 ounce (2 tablespoons) cream cheese

1 large egg, whisked

¾ cup (68 grams) pork panko (see note)

TOPPINGS:

Sauce of choice (about ½ cup)

Shredded cheese of choice (about 1 cup/4 ounces)

Pepperoni slices and/or other meat topping(s) of choice (1 to 2 ounces)

1. Preheat the oven to 425°F. Line a sheet pan with parchment paper or a silicone baking mat.

2. To make the crust, put the mozzarella, cream cheese, egg, and panko in a medium microwave-safe bowl and mix well.

3. Microwave for 90 seconds, stopping to stir in 30-second increments, until the cheese is fully melted. Continue to stir the mixture until you have a cohesive dough; as you work the dough, it will cool and start to firm up. At that point, you may want to switch to your hands to knead the dough, or you can continue working it (vigorously) with the spoon.

4. Once you have a cohesive ball of dough, place it on the prepared pan and, using your hands, spread it out to a thickness of about ¼ inch. Use a fork to poke holes all over the dough to keep it from bubbling up in the oven.

5. Bake until cooked through and lightly browned, about 10 minutes.

6. Top the crust with your favorite sauce, cheese, and meat and put back in the oven for about 8 more minutes, until the cheese is melted.

Note:

While I recommend using pork panko for this recipe, if you do not consume pork, you may replace the panko with ¼ cup Chicken Flour (page 98).

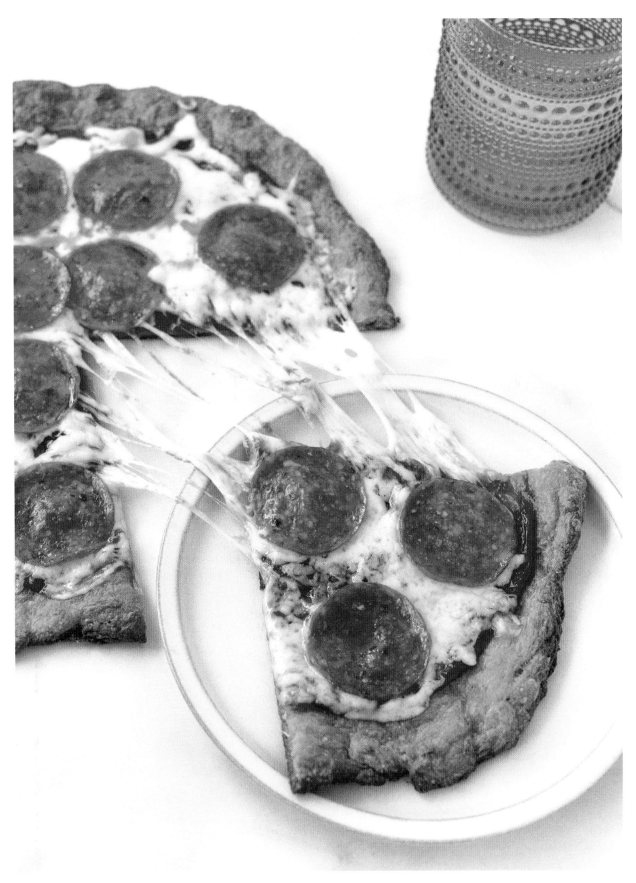

meatza

YIELD:
1 (12-inch) pizza
(2 to 4 servings)

PREP TIME:
10 minutes

COOK TIME:
35 minutes

This pork-free crust is for those of you who avoid eating piggies; it's a direct result of request after request from my community for alternatives to pork. I made the Carnizza recipe (page 182) first and loved it so much, but it's like having a second child: you love them both equally and for different reasons. I can't pick a favorite; it just depends on what ingredients I'm in the mood for. I'm sure you'll feel the same way. I highly recommend using Browned Butter Cream Sauce (page 206) as the sauce for this crust, or you can use a traditional tomato-based pizza sauce if you lean more toward a ketovore approach.

FOR THE CRUST:

1 large egg

1 pound ground chicken

¾ cup shredded mozzarella cheese (about 3 ounces)

¼ cup shredded Parmesan cheese (about ¾ ounce)

¼ teaspoon salt

TOPPINGS:

Sauce of choice (about ½ cup)

Shredded cheese of choice (about 1 cup/4 ounces)

Pepperoni slices, crumbled cooked Italian sausage, and/or other meat toppings of choice (2 to 4 ounces)

1. Preheat the oven to 400°F. Line a sheet pan with a silicone mat or parchment paper.

2. Put all the ingredients for the crust in a food processor and chop/pulse well, until the mixture is evenly combined.

3. Scrape the crust mixture onto the prepared pan. Using your hands, spread it out to a thickness of about ¼ inch.

4. Bake the crust until light brown, about 25 minutes.

5. Top the crust with your favorite sauce, cheese, and meat toppings and put back into the oven until the cheese has melted, 8 to 10 minutes.

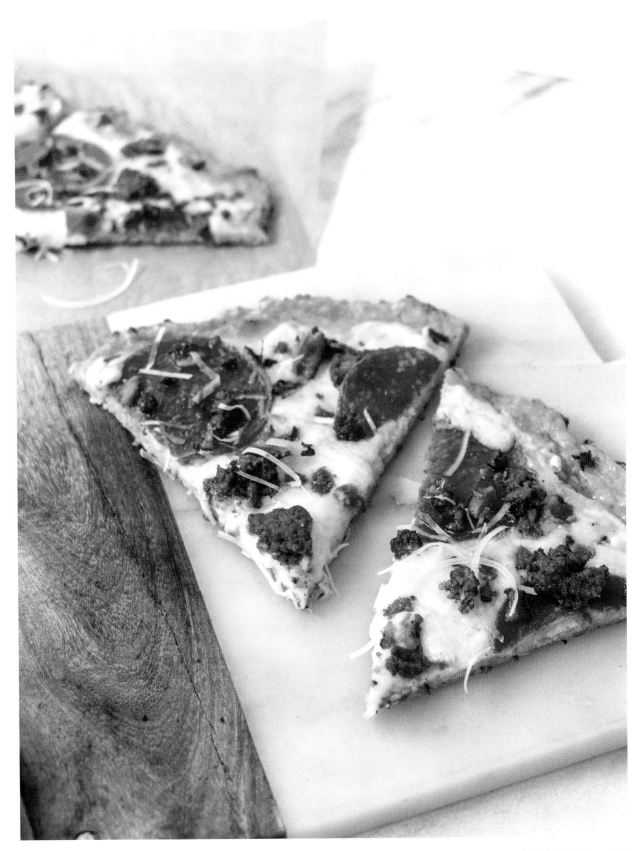

tuna melt patties

YIELD:
4 patties (2 servings)

PREP TIME:
10 minutes

COOK TIME:
6 minutes

These little guys may look like tuna cakes, but don't let their appearance fool you. They taste so much like your old favorite tuna melt sandwich, you won't even notice that there isn't any bread. You can make them in an air fryer if you prefer (see the note below), but they are so much more delicious when pan-fried in butter.

1 (5-ounce) can tuna packed in water, drained

1 large egg, whisked

¼ cup shredded cheddar cheese (about 1 ounce)

Pinch of kosher salt

1 tablespoon salted butter, for the pan

1. Put the tuna, egg, and cheese in a medium-size bowl. Season with the salt and mix well with a fork to combine the ingredients.

2. Divide the tuna mixture into 4 equal portions and shape each portion into a patty about ½ inch thick.

3. Preheat a large skillet over medium-high heat until hot but not yet smoking, about 3 minutes. Drop in the butter and swirl to coat the pan. Place the patties in the pan and pan-fry for 2 to 3 minutes, until browned on the bottom. Flip and cook for 2 to 3 minutes more, until browned on the other side. Serve immediately with a knife and fork, or let cool for a few minutes until easy to handle and eat as a handheld meal.

To cook these in an air fryer, preheat the air fryer to 400°F on the air-fry setting. Place the patties on the air fryer tray and cook for about 8 minutes, flipping them over halfway through.

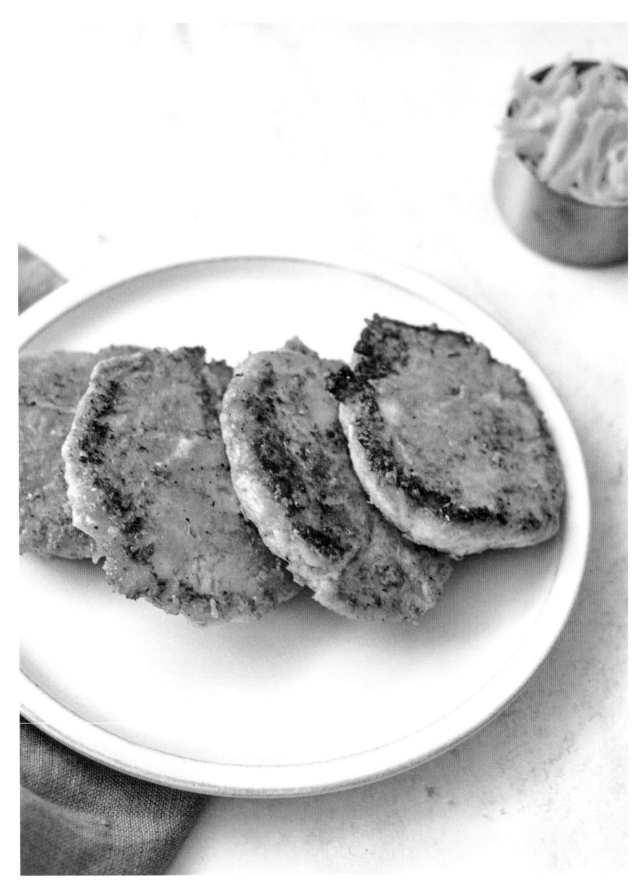

"corn" dogs

YIELD:
3 corn dogs

PREP TIME:
10 minutes

COOK TIME:
27 minutes

This recipe is one of my favorites because it evokes childhood memories. These taste like pigs in a blanket, but look like corn dogs! Traditional corn dogs are deep-fried, but in this recipe, you will be popping them in the oven. It's an easy hands-off method. Eat them as is or serve them with some mustard if you tolerate plant foods. You'll love them as much as your kids do! In fact, you may want to eat two.

FOR THE DOUGH:

1½ cups shredded mozzarella cheese (about 6 ounces)

1 ounce (2 tablespoons) cream cheese

1 large egg, whisked

¾ cup (68 grams) pork panko (see note)

3 hot dogs

1. Preheat the oven to 400°F. Line a sheet pan with parchment paper.

2. To make the dough, put the mozzarella, cream cheese, egg, and panko in a medium-size microwave-safe bowl and mix well.

3. Microwave for 90 seconds, stopping to stir in 30-second increments, until the cheese is fully melted.

4. Continue to stir the mixture until you have a cohesive dough; as you work the dough, it will cool and start to firm up. At that point, you may want to switch to your hands to knead the dough, or you can continue working it (vigorously) with the spoon.

5. Once you have a cohesive ball of dough, separate it into 3 equal portions and place them on the prepared pan. Form each portion into a ¼-inch-thick rectangle that is wide enough to wrap easily around the hot dogs and ½ inch longer on each end.

6. Place a hot dog on each dough rectangle. Wrap the dough around the hot dogs, pinching the seams and ends together to securely enclose the hot dogs.

7. Bake for 20 to 25 minutes, until deep golden brown, flipping the corn dogs over halfway through baking.

8. Allow to cool on a wire rack for a few minutes before eating to avoid burning your mouth.

Note: *While I recommend using pork panko for this recipe, if you do not consume pork, you may replace the panko with ⅓ cup Chicken Flour (page 98).*

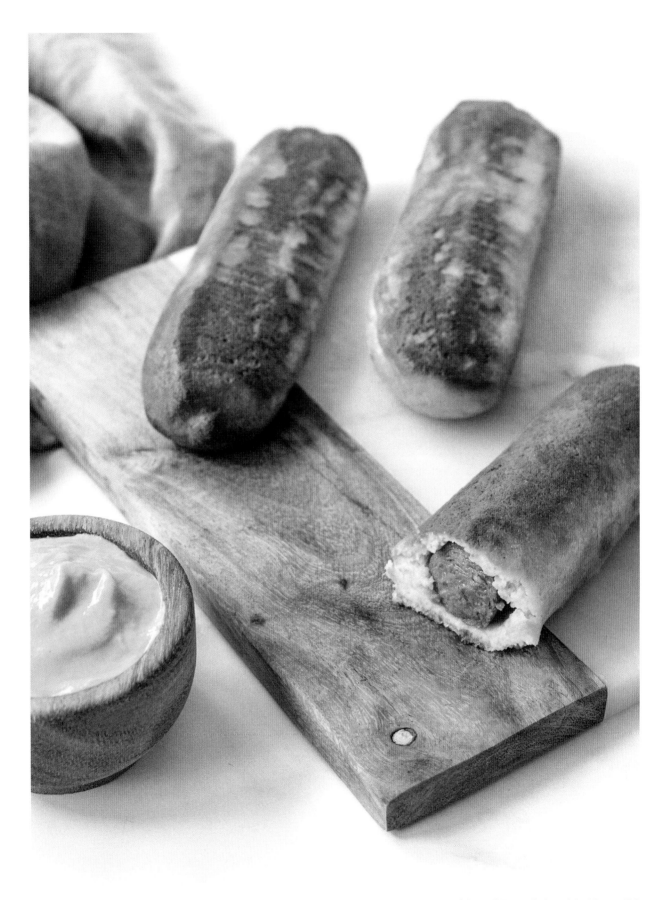

chicken nuggets

YIELD:
2 to 4 servings for adults,
4 to 6 servings for kids

PREP TIME:
10 minutes

COOK TIME:
12 minutes

What kids don't love chicken nuggies? Adults enjoy them too, and with this recipe, you don't have to worry about the (not ideal) ingredients found in the store-bought kind. I recommend cooking these nuggets on the stovetop because everything is more delicious fried in tallow, but you can also make them in an air fryer (see the note below). To stay carnivore, I dip them into sour cream, but for my kids, I also serve them with sugar-free ketchup.

1 pound boneless, skinless chicken breasts

Kosher salt

1 large egg, whisked

1½ cups pork panko

Tallow or other heat-tolerant fat of choice, for the pan

Sugar-free ketchup or sour cream, for serving (optional)

1. Cut the chicken into 1- to 2-inch chunks and salt lightly. (The pork panko will be salty, so you don't want to use too much salt.)

2. Put the whisked egg in a medium-size bowl and the panko in another medium-size bowl.

3. Heat a thin layer of tallow in a large skillet over medium-high heat.

4. Take half of the chicken pieces and place them in the bowl with the egg. Move the pieces around to completely cover them with the egg. Remove the chicken from the egg and let the excess egg drip off. Transfer the pieces to the bowl of panko and press to coat well. Set aside on a plate. Repeat with the remaining chicken pieces.

5. Working in two batches to avoid crowding, cook the breaded chicken until crispy and browned, 2 to 3 minutes, then flip and cook for another 2 to 3 minutes, until browned on both sides and cooked through. (When done, the chicken will no longer be pink in the center.) Remove the cooked chicken to a paper towel–lined plate to drain. Before cooking the remainder of the chicken, check to see that there is a thin layer of fat in the pan; if needed, add more tallow.

6. Serve the nuggets immediately with your favorite dipping sauce, if desired.

Note:

To cook the nuggets in an air fryer, preheat the air fryer to 450°F on the air-fry setting and air-fry in a basket for 10 to 15 minutes, until crispy and cooked through.

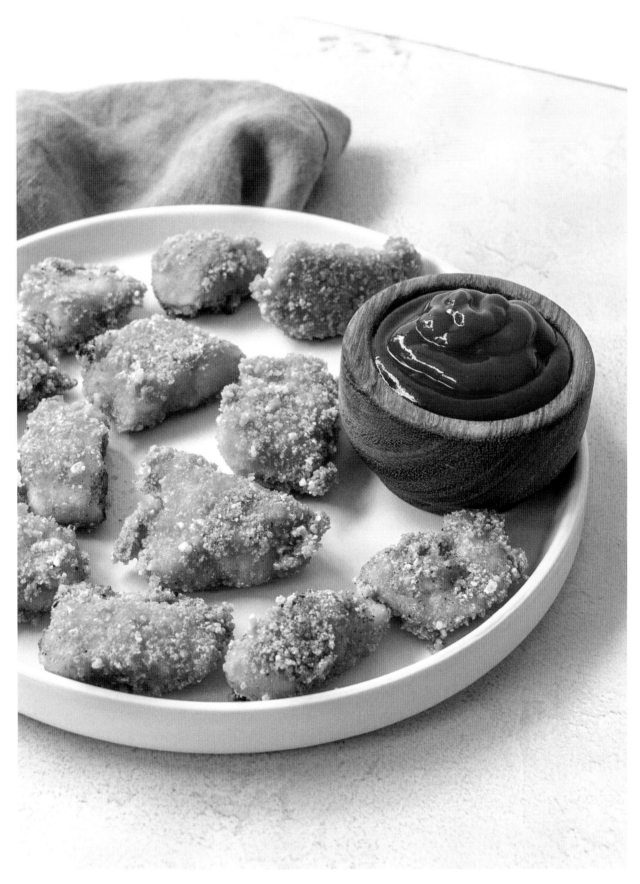

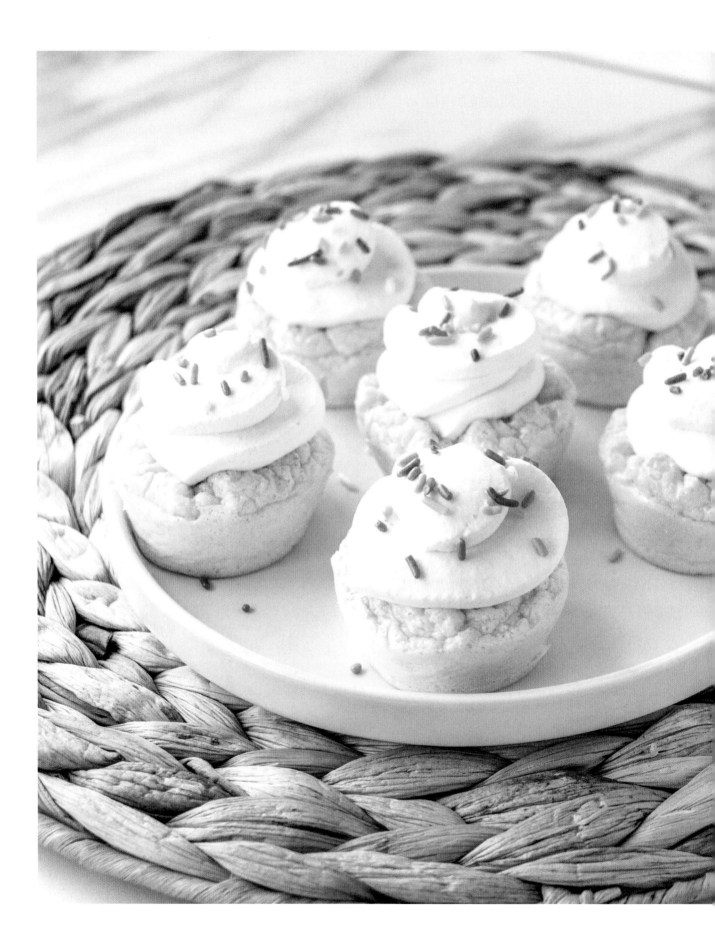

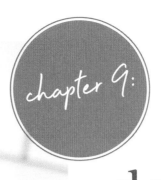

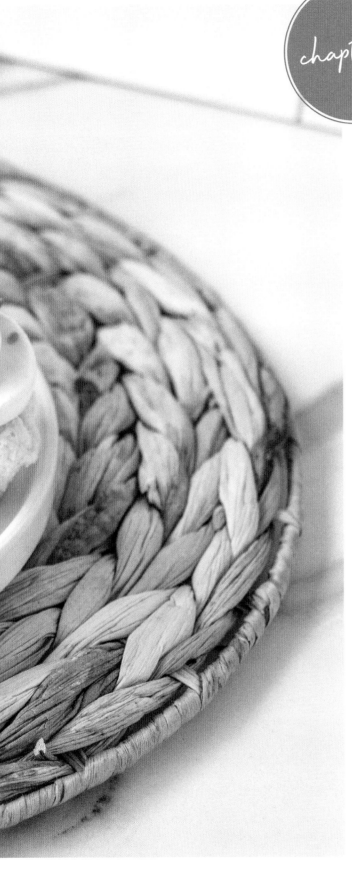

desserts

carnivore
ice cream *- 3 ways*

YIELD:
2 servings

PREP TIME:
5 minutes, plus time to churn

Ice cream is one of my favorite treats (my very favorite is coffee). I don't make it often; it's only for special occasions because it is just too good. Don't feel limited by the three flavor options listed here. The cream and yolks are the base for whichever flavors you want to create. Maybe your style of eating is more animal-based and you want to add strawberries and honey. Let your imagination run wild! If the flavor falls a little flat, try adding the tiniest pinch of salt to perk it up a bit.

FOR THE BASE:

1 cup heavy cream

2 large egg yolks

FOR VANILLA ICE CREAM:
(Makes 1½ cups)

1 teaspoon vanilla extract

Tiny pinch of kosher salt

FOR COFFEE ICE CREAM:
(Makes 1½ cups)

1 teaspoon instant coffee granules or instant espresso powder (see notes)

Tiny pinch of kosher salt

FOR CHEESECAKE ICE CREAM:
(Makes 2 cups)

3 ounces (6 tablespoons) cream cheese

½ teaspoon vanilla extract

FOR SERVING:

Freshly whipped cream

1. Put the ingredients for the base and the ingredients for the flavor you're making in a blender. Blend until well combined. If making the cheesecake flavor, make sure to blend until the mixture is smooth and there are no lumps of cream cheese remaining.

2. Pour the mixture into your ice cream maker and churn according to the manufacturer's instructions; churn time will vary, but most will take 10 to 15 minutes.

3. The finished product has the consistency of frozen yogurt, so you can serve as is, or put in the freezer for a bit to firm up.

4. Top with whipped cream and serve! Store leftover ice cream in the freezer for no longer than a month for optimal flavor. Once frozen solid, allow the ice cream to soften on the counter for a bit before scooping.

Notes: This recipe uses raw eggs. The best choice is to use farm-fresh pastured eggs from a trusted source. If you are concerned about consuming raw eggs, you can use pasteurized eggs for this recipe.

For the coffee flavor, it's important to use instant coffee granules or instant espresso powder so the coffee dissolves easily. Regular coffee/espresso grounds will not work. I also recommend using instant decaf, unless you want to be buzzing around on a caffeine high.

special equipment:
Ice cream maker

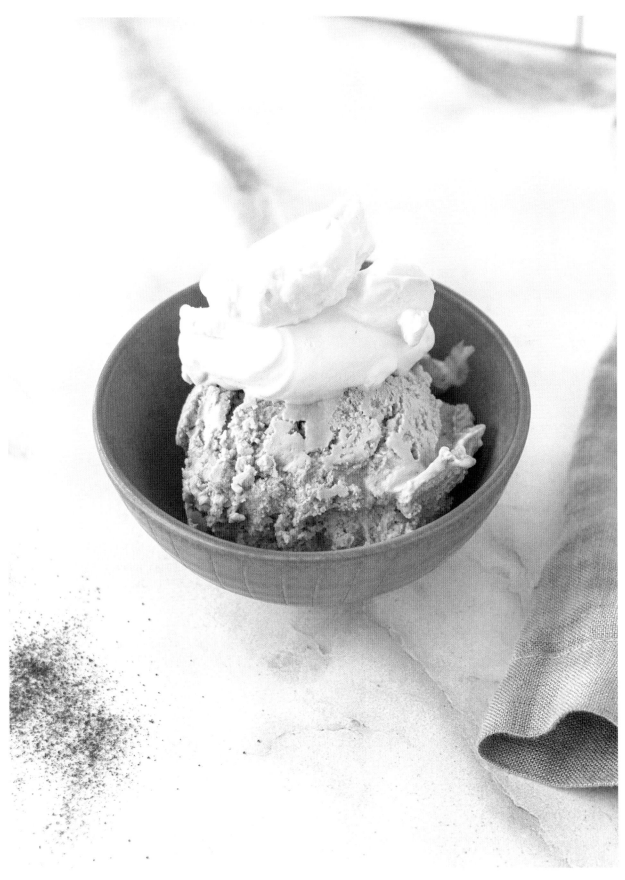

crepe cake *with* whipped cream frosting

YIELD:
1 (5-inch) cake (4 to 6 servings)

PREP TIME:
10 minutes

COOK TIME:
20 minutes

This is my go-to dessert for holidays and birthdays. It's impressive to look at, easy to prep ahead of time, and super delicious. To make this multilayer cake, you cook about a dozen crepes on the stovetop—no baking required. I prepare the crepes and whipped cream a day in advance and assemble the cake the day we are going to eat it. You can also eat the crepes as pancakes or as roll-ups with some warmed cream cheese as a filling.

FOR THE CREPE BATTER:

4 large eggs

4 ounces (½ cup) cream cheese

½ teaspoon vanilla extract (optional)

Up to 4 tablespoons (½ stick) salted butter, for the pan

FOR THE FROSTING:

1 cup heavy cream

½ teaspoon vanilla extract (optional)

1. Put the ingredients for the batter in a blender and blend until smooth. The batter will be thin.

2. Preheat a large skillet over medium heat until hot but not yet smoking.

3. Melt 1 tablespoon of the butter in the pan, then slowly pour in a small amount of batter to make two 4- to 4½-inch crepes.

4. Cook the crepes for about 2 minutes, then flip and cook for another 1 to 2 minutes, until cooked through and browned. Remove to a plate to cool.

5. Cook the rest of the crepes in batches, adding more butter as needed between batches to maintain a thin layer of fat in the pan. You should get about 12 crepes.

6. To make the frosting, whip the cream and vanilla (if using) with an electric hand mixer until soft peaks form.

7. To assemble the cake, place 4 crepes on a serving plate and spread with about 2 tablespoons of the whipped cream frosting. Place another 4 crepes on top, followed by more whipped cream. Top with the final 4 crepes, then cover the top and sides of the cake with the remaining whipped cream.

8. The cake can be eaten right away or chilled before serving.

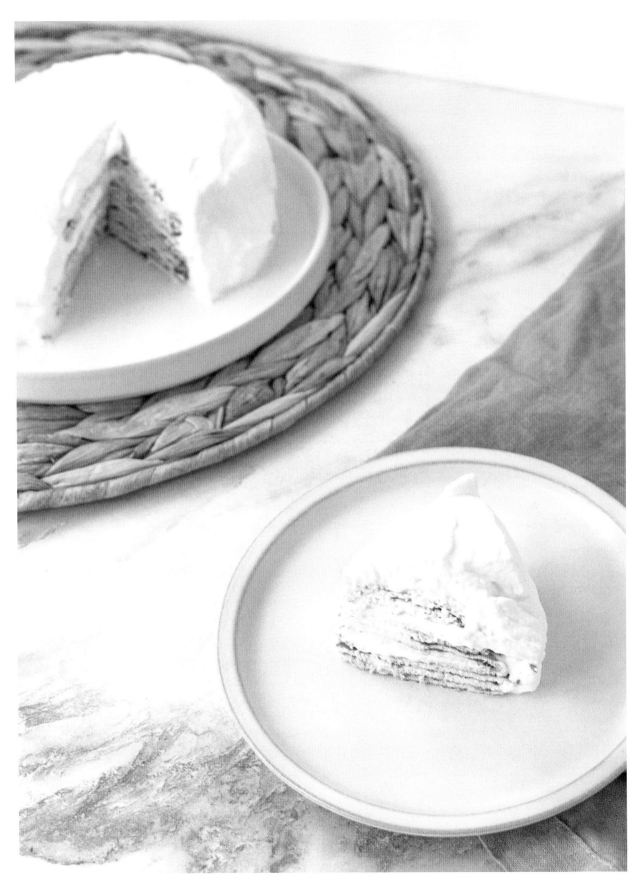

ice cream sandwiches

YIELD:
6 servings

PREP TIME:
25 minutes, plus time to chill dough (not including time to make ice cream)

COOK TIME:
15 minutes

This started out as a cookie recipe; then I thought the cookies would be even more delicious if they were frosted. And what's better than frosting? Yup, ice cream. These are great because you can make them ahead of time, pop them in the freezer, and grab one whenever you want! The ice cream is rock hard straight out of the freezer, so I suggest letting a sandwich sit out for a few minutes before you chomp into it.

FOR THE COOKIES:

¼ cup (½ stick) salted butter, softened

4 large egg yolks

2 large eggs

2 teaspoons vanilla extract

¼ cup collagen powder

1¼ cups (115 grams) pork panko

1½ teaspoons ground cinnamon

Double batch Vanilla Ice Cream (page 194) (see note)

1. In a medium-size bowl, beat the butter, egg yolks, whole eggs, and vanilla with an electric hand mixer on medium speed until blended. If there are still some tiny pieces of butter, that is OK.

2. Add the collagen and mix until it's fully incorporated, then add the panko and cinnamon and mix once more until combined.

3. Place the bowl in the freezer for about 15 minutes, until the dough is firm enough that it can be shaped without being sticky.

4. While the dough is chilling, preheat the oven to 400°F and line a sheet pan with parchment paper.

5. When the dough is firm, divide it into 12 equal pieces. Roll one piece into a ball and set it on the prepared pan. Using the palm of your hand, squish the dough into a very thin round cookie, about ¼ inch thick and 3 inches wide. Repeat with the remaining pieces of dough. The cookies will not spread during baking, so they can be closely spaced on the pan.

6. Bake until cooked through and browned on the edges, about 15 minutes. Allow to sit on the pan for a few minutes to reabsorb some of the butter that releases during baking.

7. Transfer the cookies to a wire rack to cool. Remove the ice cream from the freezer and allow it to soften so it's easy to spread.

8. Once the cookies are cool, place one-sixth (about ½ cup) of the ice cream onto a cookie, spreading it to the edges, then top with another cookie.

9. Wrap each ice cream sandwich with plastic wrap, place in a bag or container, and set in the freezer until the ice cream firms back up, about 2 hours.

10. If the ice cream sandwiches are frozen solid, let them sit out for a few minutes to soften before serving. Leftovers will keep for up to a month.

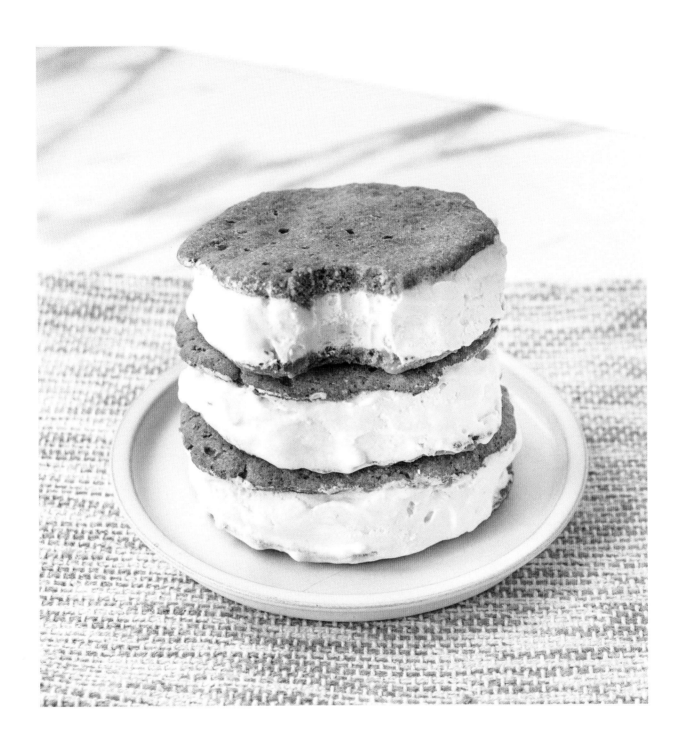

Note: To make this recipe go even faster the day of assembly, have a batch of ice cream already made. Allow it to soften a bit on the counter while the cookies are cooling. Otherwise, you can make a fresh batch of ice cream while the dough is in the freezer; that way, the ice cream will be spreadable and ready to use as is, without needing to be softened.

cheesecake mousse

YIELD:
2 cups (4 to 6 servings)

PREP TIME:
10 minutes

There's nothing like a light bite of dessert after a steak. This mousse is perfect if you have guests over because you can make it ahead of time, portion it into individual servings, and keep them in the refrigerator until you're ready to serve. Feel free to play around with the flavors, too. I think pumpkin pie spice would be delicious.

1 cup heavy cream

1 (8-ounce) package cream cheese, softened

1 teaspoon vanilla extract (optional)

½ teaspoon ground cinnamon, plus extra for garnish (optional)

1. In a medium-size bowl, whip the cream with an electric hand mixer on high speed until medium peaks form, 3 to 5 minutes. The cream should be soft and voluminous, not too firm or overmixed.

2. Put the softened cream cheese in a large bowl and add the vanilla and cinnamon, if using. Mix well with a spoon until well combined and creamy.

3. Gently fold half of the whipped cream into the cream cheese. Add the remaining whipped cream and gently stir until it is evenly incorporated.

4. Spoon or pipe the mousse into little ramekins or dessert glasses and chill before serving.

5. Garnish with a sprinkle of cinnamon, if desired.

Note: *If you have one, a stand mixer is a great option for whipping the cream in Step 1. Because it's hands-off, you can proceed with Step 2 while the cream is being whipped. If using a stand mixer, be sure to use the wire whisk attachment.*

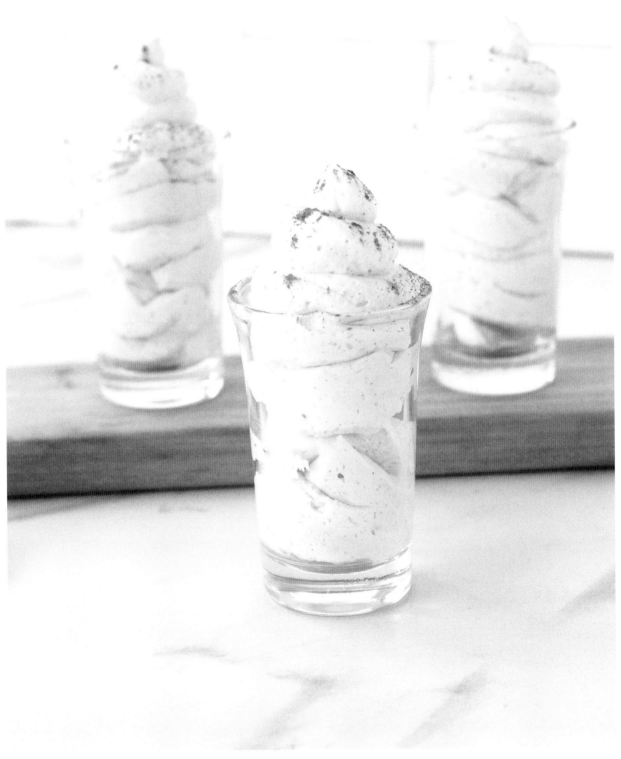

vanilla cupcakes *with* whipped cream frosting

YIELD:
12 cupcakes

PREP TIME:
15 minutes

COOK TIME:
50 minutes

These cupcakes are a spin-off of the viral cloud bread. Topped with a whipped cream frosting, they make a perfect little treat. The sprinkles are not carnivore friendly, but they are dye-free and help make this sugar-free recipe a little more fun if you are making it for kids. You can prepare the components one day ahead, store the cupcakes and frosting separately in the refrigerator, and pipe the frosting onto the cupcakes before serving.

5 large eggs, separated

⅛ teaspoon cream of tartar

5 ounces (10 tablespoons) cream cheese, softened

1½ teaspoons vanilla extract

⅛ teaspoon kosher salt

FOR THE FROSTING:

2 cups heavy cream

1 teaspoon vanilla extract

Naturally colored sprinkles, for topping (optional)

special equipment:
Standard-size 12-well silicone muffin pan

1. In a large mixing bowl, whip the egg whites and cream of tartar on high with an electric hand mixer until stiff peaks form, about 3 minutes.

2. In a small food processor or blender, blend the egg yolks, cream cheese, vanilla, and salt until smooth, then pour into a large bowl.

3. Gently fold half of the whipped whites into the cream cheese mixture, being careful not to deflate them. Repeat with the remaining whipped whites. If the two mixtures don't appear to be fully incorporated after you've folded in the whites, use the hand mixer on low for about 10 seconds to ensure all is mixed very well and smooth, being careful not to compromise the fluffiness of the mixture.

4. Generously fill the wells of the muffin pan with the batter; use about ⅓ cup of batter per well, depending on the exact size of your pan. The batter should go to the very top of the wells, to the point of overflowing. That's OK, because the cupcakes will not expand as they bake.

5. Bake until lightly browned on top, 45 to 50 minutes. When done, a toothpick will come out clean when inserted in the middle of a cupcake.

6. Let cool in the pan on a wire rack. While the cupcakes are cooling, make the frosting.

7. Using the mixer, beat the heavy cream and vanilla on high speed until soft peaks form, 2 to 3 minutes.

8. Transfer the frosting to a piping bag (or a plastic bag with one corner cut off) and pipe onto the cooled cupcakes.

9. Store any leftovers in the refrigerator for up to 3 days.

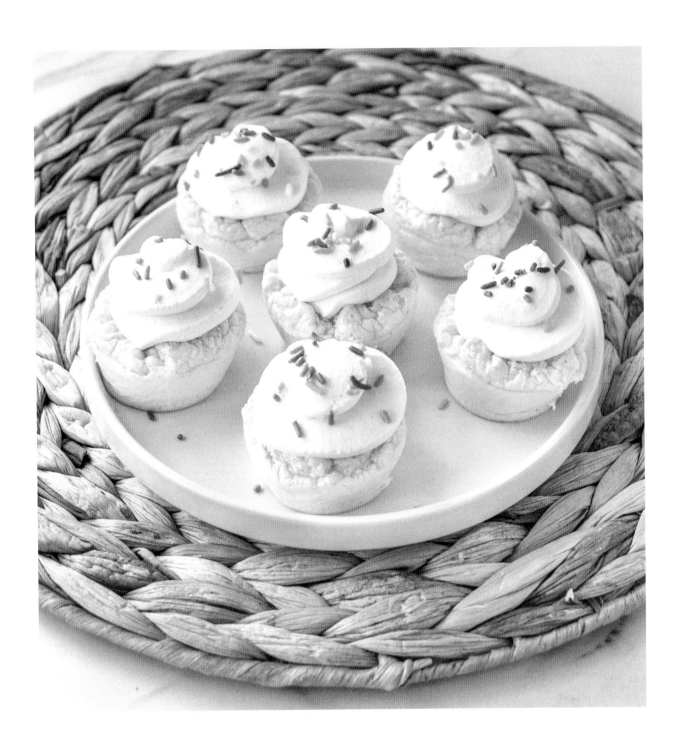

Notes: If you have one, a stand mixer is a great option for Step 1 of this recipe. Because it's hands-off, you can proceed with Step 2 while the egg whites are being whipped. If using a stand mixer, be sure to use the wire whisk attachment.

To ensure the baked cupcakes release easily from the pan, it's important to blend the two batter mixtures together fully and evenly (per Step 3) and to fully bake the cupcakes (per Step 5).

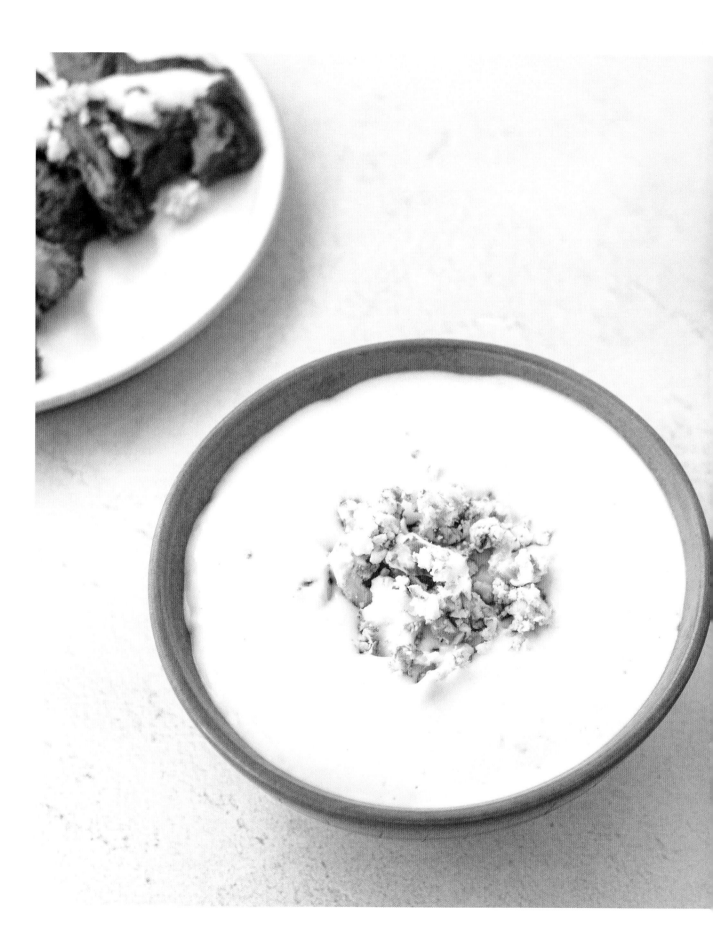

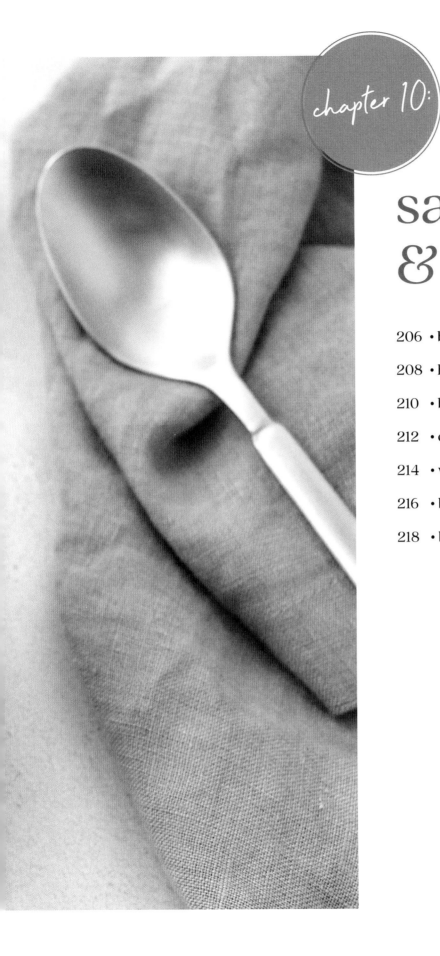

chapter 10:

sauces
& dips

browned butter cream sauce

YIELD:
About 1¾ cups (4 to 6 servings)

PREP TIME:
5 minutes

COOK TIME:
15 minutes

I must refrain from eating this sauce by the spoonful, like it's a soup. It's just that delicious! The basis of this recipe is a classic Alfredo sauce, but with the added step of browning the butter. It gives the sauce a unique nutty, almost caramel-like flavor, and you can't go wrong when you mix that with cream and Parmesan. Pour this sauce over either Panko Noodles (page 92) or Egg White Noodles (page 94), pair it with grilled chicken, or simply go at it with a spoon. You're in for a decadent meal.

½ cup (1 stick) salted butter

1 cup heavy cream

2 cups shredded Parmesan cheese (about 8 ounces)

1. Melt the butter in a medium-size saucepan over medium heat. After it melts, continue to cook it, stirring frequently, until it has browned, about 5 minutes. It will develop a nutty, caramel-like aroma. Be careful not to let it burn, which can happen quickly after it starts to change to a golden color.

2. As soon as the butter has browned, pour in the cream and warm it for 2 minutes.

3. After the cream is warmed, add the cheese. Whisk until it is melted and the sauce is smooth, 1 to 2 minutes.

Note: *If making a half batch of this recipe for the Standard Carnivore Meal Plan (page 46), use a small saucepan in Step 1.*

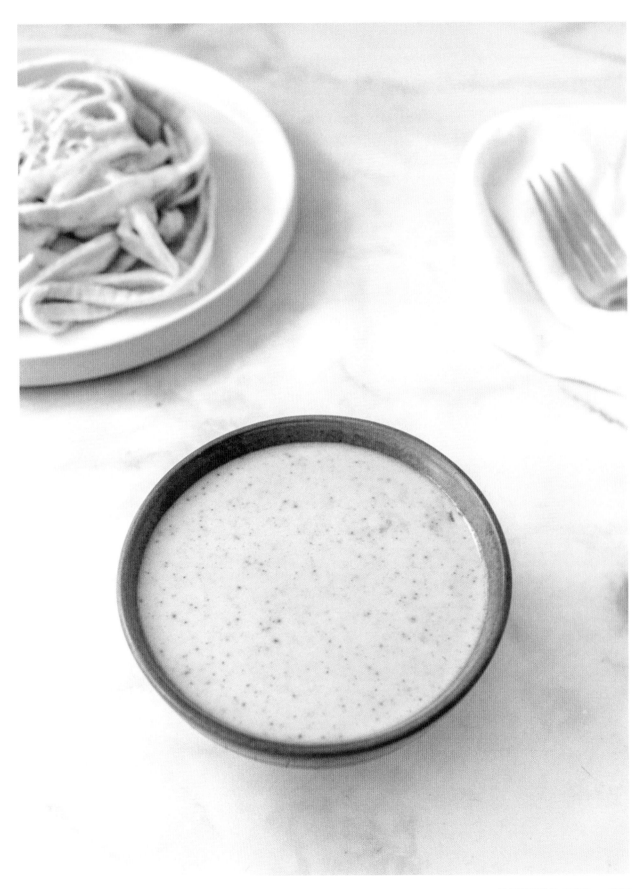

hollandaise sauce

YIELD:
About ¾ cup (4 servings)

PREP TIME:
10 minutes

This classic sauce is used in Eggs Benedict (page 62), but you can pour it on everything. You can even use it cold as a buttery mayo! Try it in place of mayonnaise when making Instant Pot Deviled Eggs (page 110)—so delicious! I recommend including the lemon juice if you tolerate it. The tang it adds really brings this sauce to life.

4 large egg yolks

1 tablespoon lemon juice

½ cup (1 stick) salted butter, melted

1. Put the egg yolks in a blender (or, if using an immersion blender, put the yolks in a tall mug or wide-mouth mason jar).

2. Add the lemon juice to the yolks and blend until combined.

3. Slowly add the melted butter to the yolk mixture while continuing to blend until thickened and smooth.

4. Serve immediately or keep warm for up to 2 hours before serving. To keep the sauce warm, you can transfer it to a thermos or simply store it, covered, at the back of your stove.

5. Store leftover sauce in the refrigerator for up to 4 days. To rewarm it, gently heat it either in the microwave, stirring every 15 seconds, or in a saucepan. You may need to reblend it if it separates.

Note: *This recipe uses raw eggs. The best choice is to use farm-fresh pastured eggs from a trusted source. If you are concerned about consuming raw eggs, you can use pasteurized eggs for this recipe.*

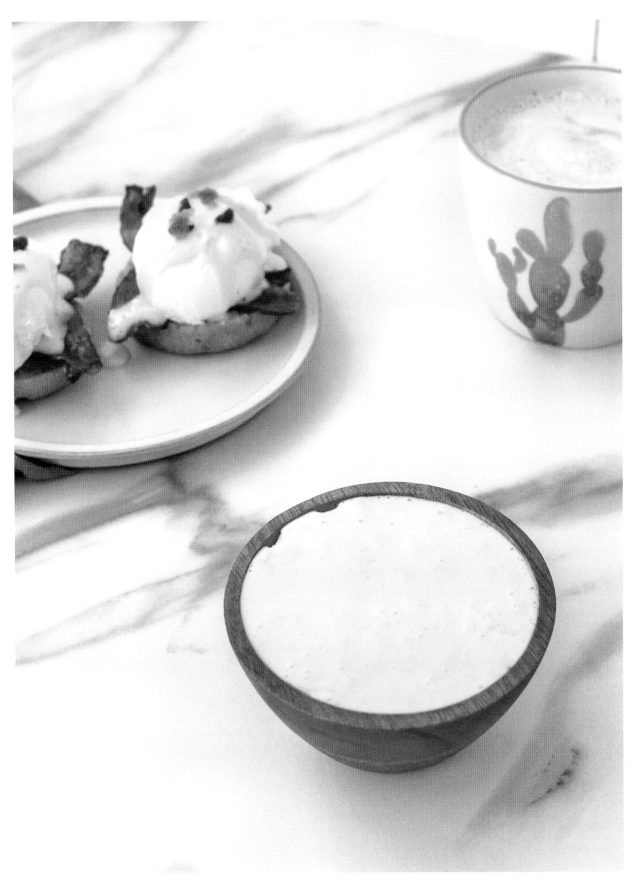

butter bacon mayonnaise

YIELD:
About 1 cup (6 to 8 servings)

PREP TIME:
7 minutes

This is a healthier alternative to store-bought mayonnaise because it is made from butter and bacon grease instead of seed oils. Use it as a sandwich spread or in Instant Pot Deviled Eggs (page 110), or dollop it on a burger. You can leave out the mustard and lemon juice if you do not tolerate them, but they lend a delicious zing to this sauce.

½ cup (1 stick) salted butter, softened

¼ cup bacon grease (see notes)

4 large egg yolks

1 teaspoon Dijon mustard (optional)

1 teaspoon lemon juice (optional)

1. Put all the ingredients in a mini food processor or blender. Blend until nicely whipped. Serve immediately.

2. Store leftover mayo in an airtight container in the refrigerator for up to 4 days. The mayo sets up when it gets cold, so let it soften a bit before using.

I keep bacon grease on the counter, so the texture is always nice and soft. If you store your bacon grease in the fridge, allow it to soften at room temperature before making this recipe.

This recipe uses raw eggs. The best choice is to use farm-fresh pastured eggs from a trusted source. If you are concerned about consuming raw eggs, you can use pasteurized eggs for this recipe.

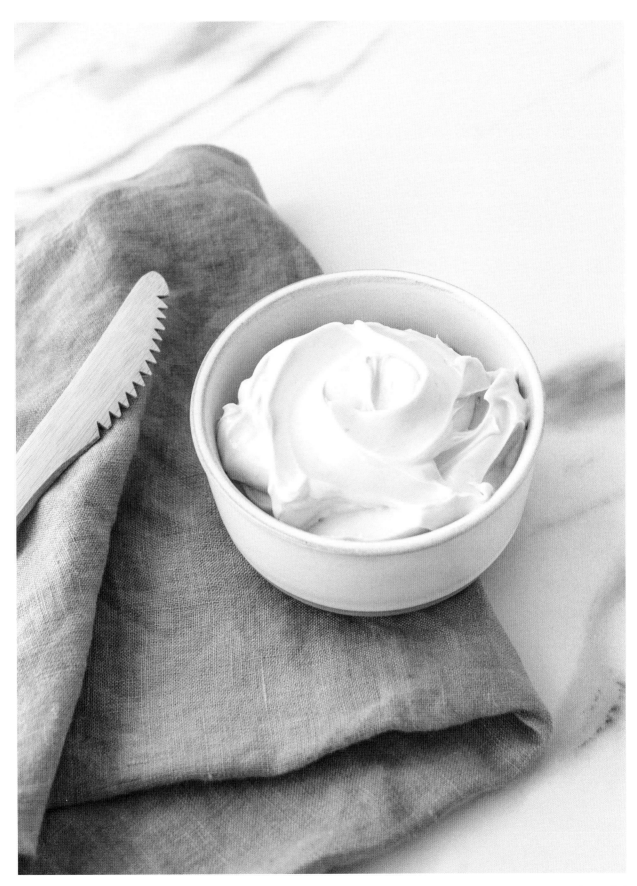

creamy feta dip

YIELD:
About 1¼ cups (6 to 8 servings)

PREP TIME:
10 minutes

This dip is very versatile! It's wonderful as is, but you can make it your own. Want it tangier? Ditch the cream cheese and add more yogurt. Don't have cream cheese on hand? Add some heavy cream instead. Wanna get wild? Add a squeeze of lemon juice. I recommend serving this dip with Kofta Meatballs (page 162) or Lamb Lollipops (page 164), but it's also perfect for Meat Chips (page 108) or as a spread for burgers or a topping for grilled chicken breast to bump up the fat content.

½ cup plain Greek yogurt

3 ounces feta cheese

2 ounces (¼ cup) cream cheese, softened

Put all the ingredients in a mini food processor or blender and blend until smooth and creamy. Serve cold or at room temperature.

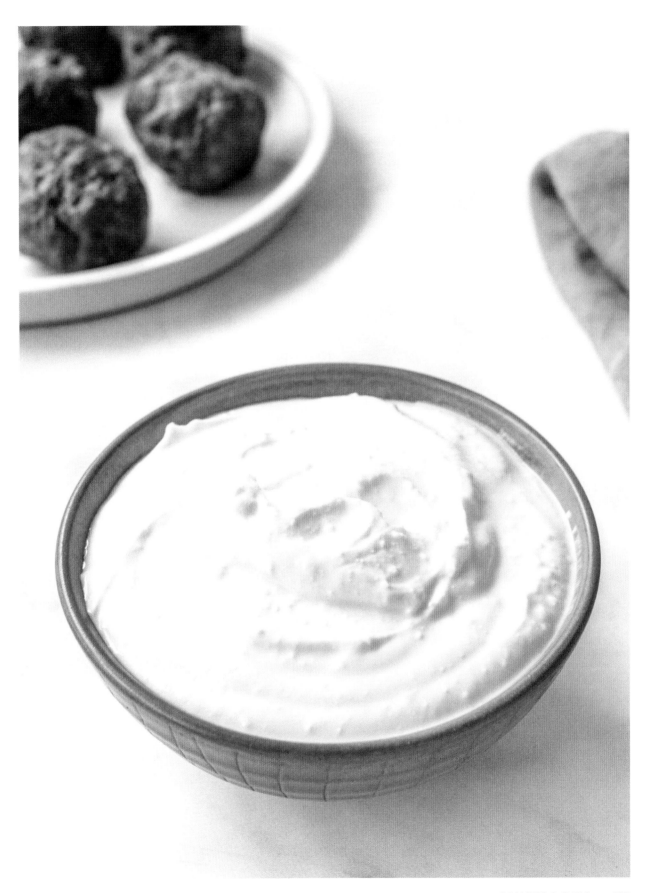

whipped goat cheese dip

YIELD:
About 1 cup (6 to 8 servings)

PREP TIME:
5 minutes

This dip is great served with your favorite meat chips (see page 27 for a store-bought suggestion or page 108 for my recipe), some crispy Baked Bacon (page 166), or on top of a bacon burger. But it's also OK if you just eat it with a spoon.

1 (4-ounce) log fresh (soft) goat cheese

2 ounces (¼ cup) cream cheese, softened

¼ cup heavy cream

Put all the ingredients in a mini food processor or blender and blend until smooth and creamy. Serve cold or at room temperature.

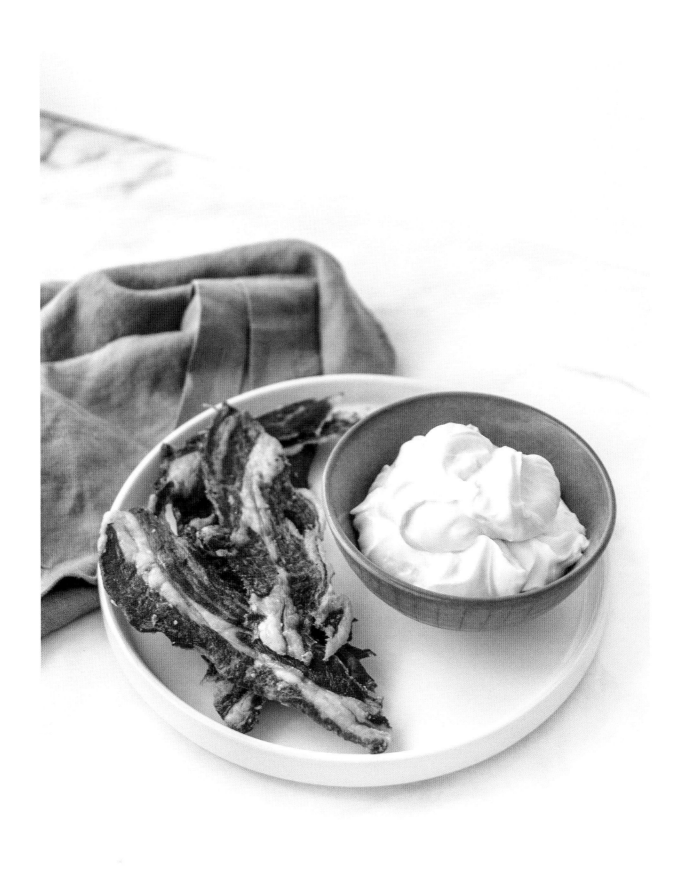

blue cheese cream sauce

YIELD:
About 1 cup (4 to 6 servings)

PREP TIME:
5 minutes

COOK TIME:
5 minutes

This sauce is fabulous on all the things, especially when served warm and poured over a rib eye or skirt steak (see pages 150 and 152, respectively). I even love it cold, straight from the fridge, scooped onto a hot burger patty. And for the wild plant eaters in your life: if you caramelize some onions in the pan before pouring in the cream, they'll be in heaven.

½ cup heavy cream

1¼ cups crumbled blue cheese (about 5 ounces), plus extra for garnish if desired

1. Pour the cream into a small saucepan and set over medium-low heat.

2. Once the cream is warm, add the cheese and whisk occasionally until it is melted and the sauce has thickened, about 5 minutes.

3. Serve warm, garnished with crumbled blue cheese, if desired.

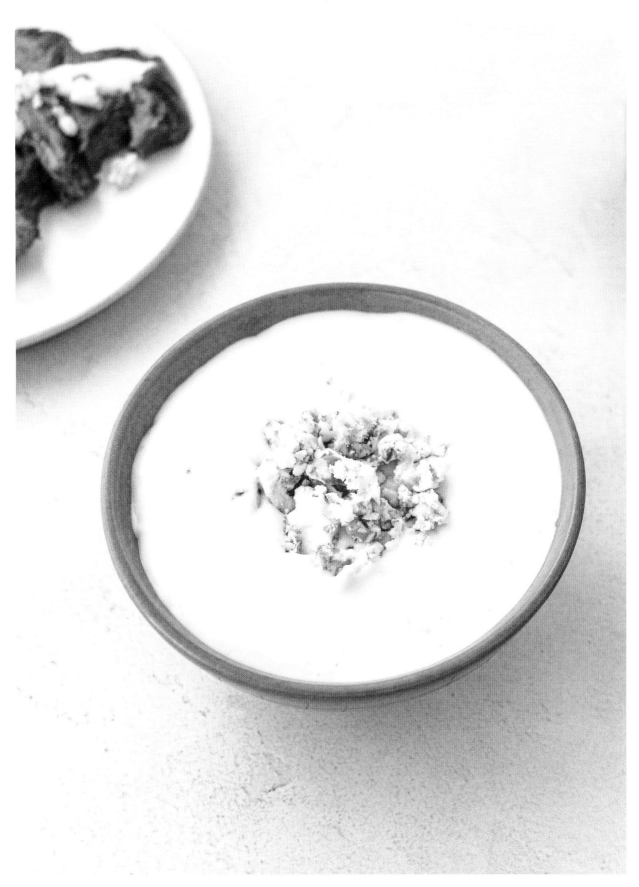

bacon-infused sandwich spread

YIELD:
About 1 cup (6 to 8 servings)

PREP TIME:
10 minutes

This is a great burger topping or sandwich spread. Use one of my Tortillas (page 88) to make a wrap with your favorite deli meat, bacon, cheese, and this delicious spread for an easy ready-to-go lunch. You can also use it as a dip for meat chips, as shown.

4 ounces (½ cup) cream cheese, softened

½ cup sour cream

¼ cup Butter Bacon Mayonnaise (page 210)

Kosher salt

1. Put all the ingredients in a mini food processor or small blender and mix well.

2. Add salt to taste and serve cold. Store leftover spread in the refrigerator for up to 4 days.

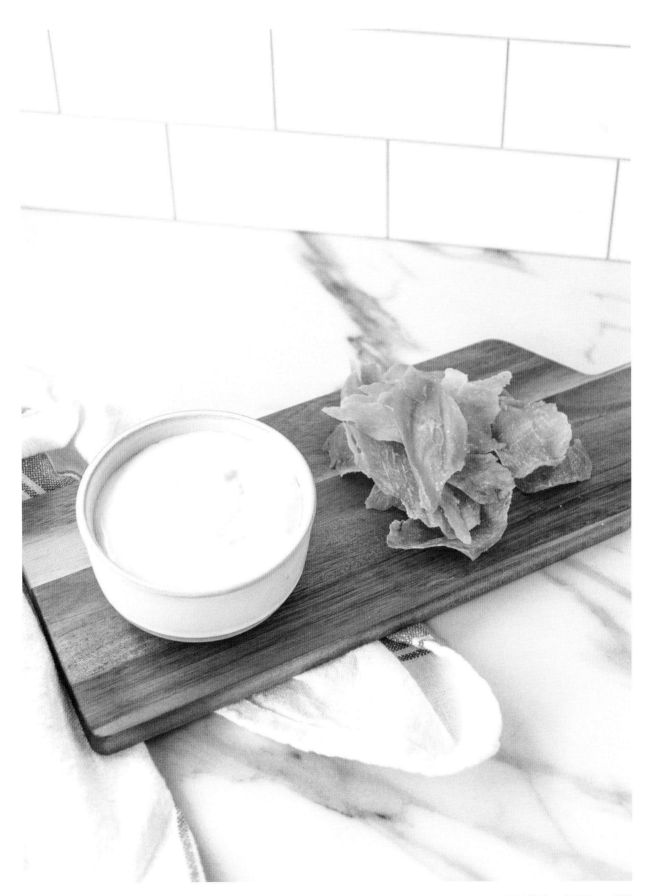

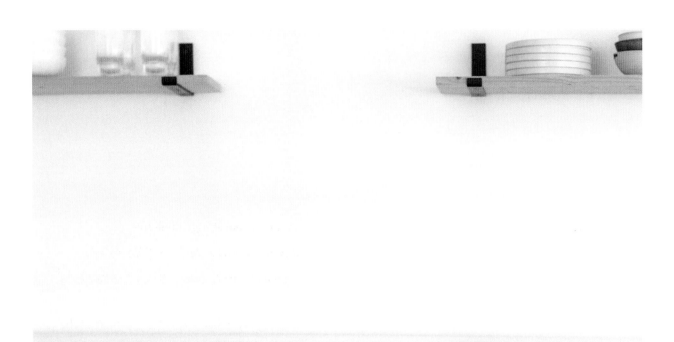

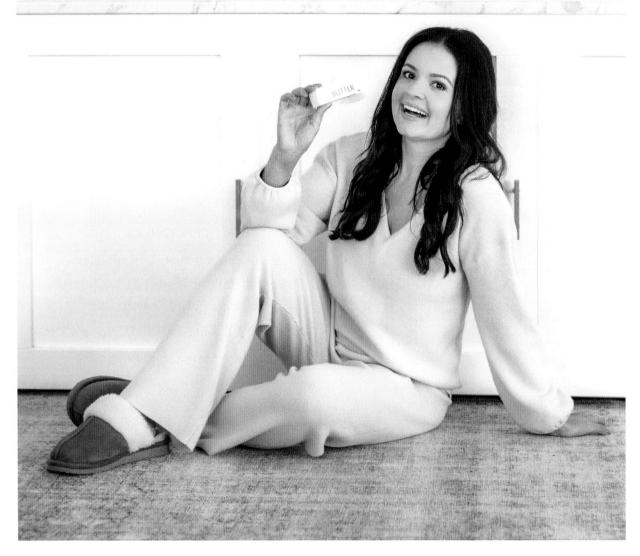

for further reading

The following is a list of experts in the carnivore diet space. Most of them also offer coaching services for additional support:

Rina Ahluwalia: YouTube @5MinuteBody

Dr. Shawn Baker: Author of *The Carnivore Diet*, YouTube @ShawnBakerMD

Dr. Ken Berry: Author of *Lies My Doctor Told Me*, YouTube @KenDBerryMD

Dr. Anthony Chaffee: YouTube @AnthonyChaffeeMD

Judy Cho: Author of *Carnivore Cure* and *The Complete Carnivore Diet for Beginners*, YouTube @NutritionwithJudy

Dani Conway: nutritionthenaturalway.com, YouTube @NTNW1

Bronson Dant: YouTube @Coach.Bronson

Sarah Franklin: inthebuffwellness.com, YouTube @InTheBuffWellness

Natalie Grasso: nataliejgrasso.com, YouTube @KetoBikiniSecrets

Jessica Henrard: thejessicatreatment.com, YouTube @TheJessicaTreatment

Kelly Hogan: YouTube @MyZeroCarbLife

Michelle Hurn: Author of *The Dietitian's Dilemma*, Instagram @RunEatMeatRepeat

Britt James: healtheditbybrittcoaching.as.me, Instagram @healtheditbybritt

Lillie Kane: YouTube @LillieKane

Professor Bart Kay: YouTube @Bart-Kay

Dr. Robert Kiltz: Author of *The Fertile Feast*, YouTube @DoctorKiltz

Bella Ma (aka Steak and Butter Gal): YouTube @SteakandButterGal

Serena Musick: purelytallow.com, YouTube @CarnivoreRevolution

Sally Norton: Author of *Toxic Superfoods*, YouTube @SKNorton

Dr. Philip Ovadia: Author of *Stay Off My Operating Table*, YouTube @IFixHearts

Mikhaila Peterson: YouTube @Mikhaila

Dr. Paul Saladino: Author of *The Carnivore Code*, YouTube @PaulSaladinoMD

Linda Salant: YouTube @TheCarnitarianLife

Dr. Sabrina Solt: stemcelltherapypro.com, YouTube @carnivoreh3

Laura Spath: YouTube @LauraSpath

Dr. Lisa Wiedeman: YouTube @CarnivoreDoctor

Jen Winkler: jenwinkler.me, YouTube @CoachJenWinkler

recipe index

breakfast

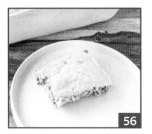
BREAKFAST CASSEROLE

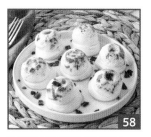
INSTANT POT BACON AND GRUYÈRE EGG BITES

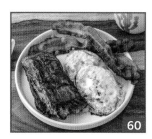
BREAKFAST OF CHAMPIONS

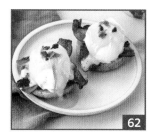
EGGS BENEDICT

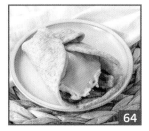
BREAKFAST BURRITO

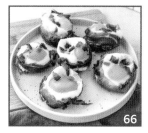
PROSCIUTTO EGG CUPS

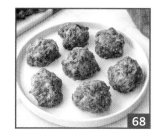
BREAKFAST MEATBALLS

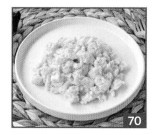
COTTAGE CHEESE EGGS

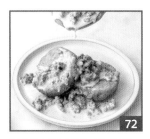
BISCUITS AND GRAVY

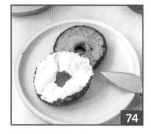
MINI BAGELS

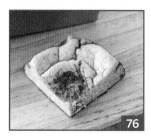
DUTCH BABY SOUFFLÉ

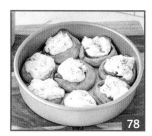
CINNAMON ROLLS

breads, wraps & noodles

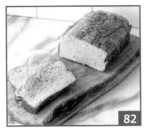
CARNIVORE BREAD

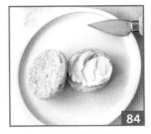
ENGLISH MUFFINS

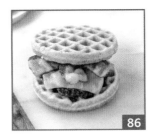
ALL-PURPOSE WAFFLES

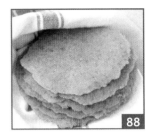
TORTILLAS

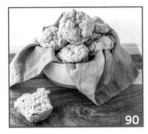
CORNBREAD MUFFINS

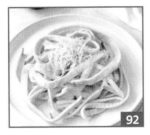
PANKO NOODLES

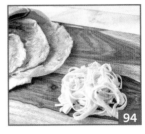
EGG WHITE NOODLES OR WRAPS

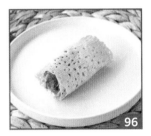
CHEESE WRAP

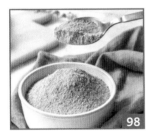
CHICKEN FLOUR

appetizers, soups & salads

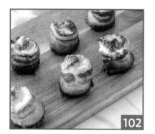
PIGGY BITES

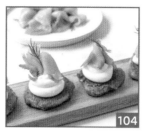
SMOKED SALMON BLINIS

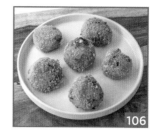
FRIED GOAT CHEESE BALLS

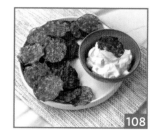
MEAT CHIPS

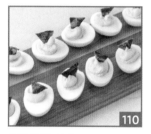
INSTANT POT DEVILED EGGS

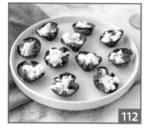
SALAMI CUPS

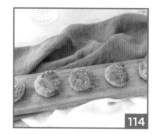
FRIED EGG YOLKS

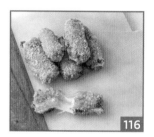
MOZZARELLA STICKS

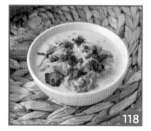
BACON CHEESEBURGER SOUP

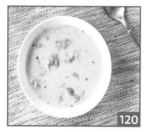
CREAMY SAUSAGE SOUP

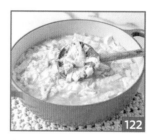
CHICKEN NOODLE SOUP

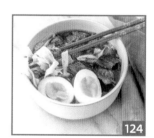
RAMEN

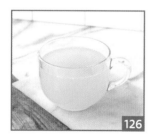
SIPPING BONE BROTH

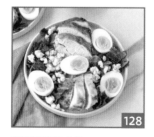
COBB SALAD

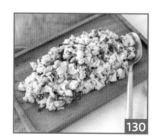
CHICKEN SALAD

simply meat

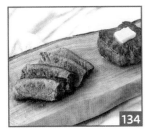
FILET MIGNON 134

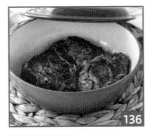
POT ROAST 136

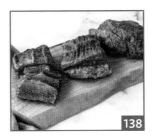
INSTANT POT SMOKED BRISKET 138

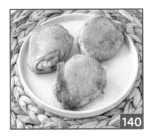
CRISPY CHICKEN THIGHS 140

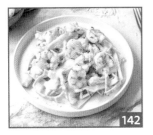
AIR FRYER SHRIMP 142

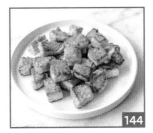
SALMON BITES 144

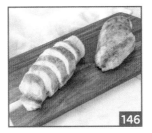
PAN-SEARED CHICKEN BREAST 146

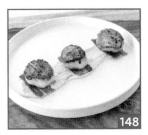
PAN-SEARED SCALLOPS 148

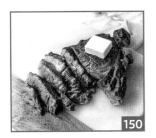
PAN-SEARED RIB EYE 150

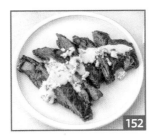
PAN-SEARED SKIRT STEAK 152

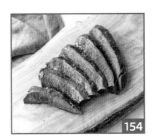
PAN-SEARED HEART 154

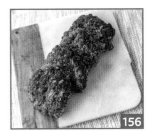
HIDDEN LIVER BURGERS 156

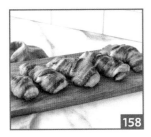
BACON-WRAPPED CHICKEN THIGHS 158

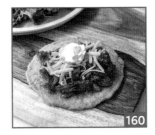
CARNITAS 160

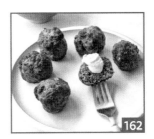
KOFTA MEATBALLS 162

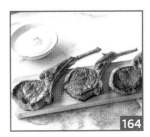
LAMB LOLLIPOPS 164

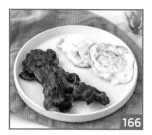

BAKED BACON

comforting classics

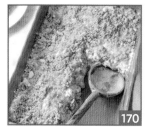

CREAMY CHICKEN
CASSEROLE WITH
CRUNCHY PANKO
TOPPING

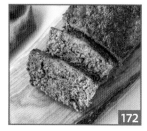

MEATLOAF

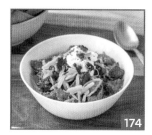

CHILI

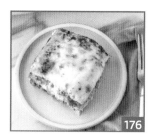

WHITE LASAGNA

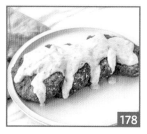

COUNTRY-FRIED STEAK
WITH GRAVY

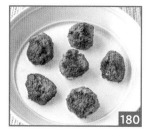

SWEDISH MEATBALLS

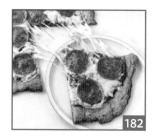

CARNIZZA

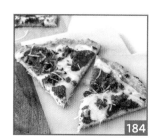

MEATZA

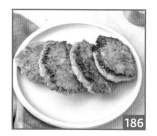

TUNA MELT PATTIES

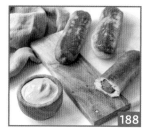

"CORN" DOGS

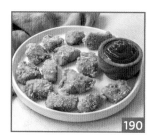

CHICKEN NUGGETS

desserts

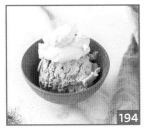
CARNIVORE ICE CREAM—3 WAYS

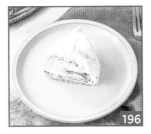
CREPE CAKE WITH WHIPPED CREAM FROSTING

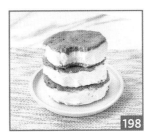
ICE CREAM SANDWICHES

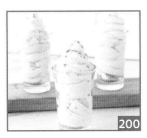
CHEESECAKE MOUSSE

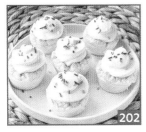
VANILLA CUPCAKES WITH WHIPPED CREAM FROSTING

sauces & dips

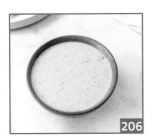
BROWNED BUTTER CREAM SAUCE

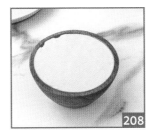
HOLLANDAISE SAUCE

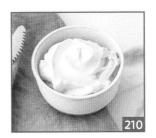
BUTTER BACON MAYONNAISE

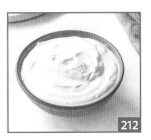
CREAMY FETA DIP

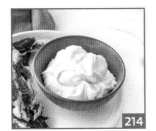
WHIPPED GOAT CHEESE DIP

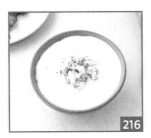
BLUE CHEESE CREAM SAUCE

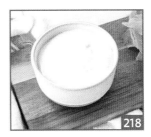
BACON-INFUSED SANDWICH SPREAD

general index

C